Do-It-Yourself
SHIATSU

How to Perform the Ancient Japanese Art of "Acupuncture without Needles"

By
Wataru Ohashi
Edited by Vicki Lindner

Mr. Ohashi is director and principal instructor of the Ohashi Institute, a nonprofit educational organization located in New York City. He and his Certified Ohashiatsu® Instructors teach his own system of technique, exercise, and meditation in many cities in the United States and Europe. If you would like to receive a list of centers and courses, please write to the Ohashi Institute at:

12 West 27th Street
Floor 9
New York, NY 10001
(Tel: 212-684-4190)

Do-It-Yourself
SHIATSU
How to Perform the Ancient Japanese Art of "Acupuncture without Needles"

By
Wataru Ohashi
Edited by Vicki Lindner

A Dutton Paperback

E. P. Dutton   **New York**

1-212-725-1818

" Path way"- газета

To my mother

I would like to thank Martha Murphy, Deborah Goodman, and Linda Schneider, who helped in the writing of this book; Jo Pizzino, Ivan Nagy and Jenny Auspos, who modeled for the photographs; and Mamoru Tanaka and Katsu Takahashi, who took these photographs. I greatly appreciate all my American friends who have helped me.

Published in the United States by E. P. Dutton,
a division of NAL Penguin Inc.,
2 Park Avenue, New York, N.Y. 10016

Published simultaneously in Canada by Fitzhenry & Whiteside Limited, Toronto

ISBN: 0-525-48312-8

Library of Congress Cataloging-in-Publication Data
Ohashi, Wataru.
  Do-it-yourself shiatsu.
  1. Shiatsu. I. Title
RM723.S503 1976   615′.822   75-29487

Contents

1. Introduction

What Is Shiatsu?

In Japanese the word *shi* means finger and *atsu* means pressure. *Shiatsu,* also called Acupressure, is an Oriental massage in which the fingers are pressed on particular points of the body to ease aches, pains, tension, fatigue, and symptoms of disease. These points are called *tsubo* and they are the specific places in the body's skin and muscular system where nerves hurt or feel uncomfortable when the flow of energy through the body is blocked. In Shiatsu we manipulate the tsubo, which sometimes initially pains the patient, but eventually starts the energy circulating again to relieve pain. The aching tsubo, however, is not the same spot as the source of complaint and may, in fact, be far away from the discomfort the patient is feeling. For example, to ease a headache we can apply pressure and stimulation in the legs and arms. To relieve the pain of hemorrhoids we stimulate the tsubo on top of the head.

The 361 tsubos, also called Acupuncture points and pressure points, are located along the "meridian lines," the fourteen channels through which the body's energy flows. These channels are invisible, but according to Oriental philosophy, exist as surely and definably as the nerves. In fact, the Shiatsu patient is sometimes conscious of a surge of energy through these lines while he or she is being manipulated. The same meridians pass through many parts of the body and connect the vital organs, which is why a "long-distance treatment," or pressing a tsubo far from the origin of the complaint, is effective. In actual practice we use only about ninety-two tsubos in Shiatsu. The acupuncturist inserts his needles at the same points.

Like Acupuncture, Shiatsu, when performed skillfully, can relieve many kinds of chronic problems and disabling aches and pains. Many of my patients are dancers, often apt to injure muscles and tendons while they work. If a dancer is injured and can't appear in a scheduled performance, he loses not only money, but a great deal of status and credibility. Ivan Nagy, the great international dancer with the American Ballet Theatre, injured himself and was told by his doctor not to perform. He came to me and I gave him Shiatsu for an hour. By the next morning he was dancing again. His fellow performers could not believe what they saw. A woman, a Yoga teacher, had been suffering with extreme constipation for two weeks. Her cramps were terrible. After one Shiatsu treatment she found relief. When a friend of mine has a cold, I give him Shiatsu. Colds usually create a lot of tension in the back. Shiatsu can relieve this symptom and make the patient feel more comfortable.

Ideally, Shiatsu is best used not to cure disease but to maintain health, vitality, and stamina in the body, to strengthen the internal organs and prevent energy from getting blocked in the tsubo to begin with. Even as a beginner you will find Shiatsu very effective in relieving the external symptoms of many diseases as well as simple muscular aches and pains caused by tension and fatigue. Although a professional will often combine Shiatsu with other forms of Oriental medicine to completely *cure* disease, as a beginner you should never try to cure disease with Shiatsu alone. Always consult a doctor if you suspect a friend is seriously ill; be sure to follow the precautions I give in chapter 3 and the chapters dealing with specific parts of the body. In general, you will find Shiatsu most useful in raising the life energy level of your friend to make him strong, healthy, and resistant to disease. You can also give yourself Shiatsu and do a series of exercises to make your own body stronger, which I have developed in the course of my own training. *Never* equate your status as an amateur with that of a professional practitioner of Oriental medicine.

The Body from the Eastern Point of View

In ancient civilizations there was no discipline called science from which answers to questions about nature and the universe could be derived. As far as people knew, there existed only the earth and everything around it. In the Orient a cosmology evolved which views all natural phenomena as divided first into the physical compositions of plant, heat, earth, mineral, or liquid, then into the five natural elements of wood, metal, water, fire, and earth. All phenomena are also thought to be divided into two other categories, or energy forces: the Yin, or negative, and the Yang, or positive. Women are considered Yin, or passive, and men Yang, or active. The interplay of these two forces and the ways in which they mutate from one to the other are thought necessary for all function and change in the universe.

In the Orient the human body is regarded as a microcosm of the natural universe and therefore governed by the five elements and the forces of Yin and Yang. The organs of the body, too, are divided into interdependent groups of six *Fu* (or Yang, positive) and six *Zo* (or Yin, negative) organs, each of which also represents one of the five elements and works together with another, complementary organ. (For example, the small intestine complements the heart; the liver complements the gall bladder, which collects liver bile.) If the heart, a fire organ, is injured, the liver, a wood organ, would be damaged too, since fire can destroy wood. Treatment of disease, too, must complement the damaged organ or body part. The energy system connecting the organs is the meridian line system, which is a combination of horizontal and vertical channels of energy. Shiatsu improves the flow of energy through this system, which I will explain at length in chapter 2.

Origins of Shiatsu

It is easy to imagine how the art of Shiatsu came into existence, just by considering your own experience with pain or discomfort. The natural reaction to pain is to place the hand on the area that hurts you, or to press it with your fingers. If you have a sinus headache you squeeze your nose. If you feel tense and nervous you rub your neck. If your stomach hurts you rub or clutch it. A mother instinctively rubs and caresses a baby when it begins to cry. Animals soothe themselves and each other by stimulation with the tongue. Shiatsu is merely an established, concrete, and more complex method of this instinctual form of healing.

In early times kings, saints, and clergy were believed to possess God-given powers not belonging to common men. Both in the West and in the Orient this power, usually communicated through touch, was used to heal. Professional healers, too, were thought to possess this divine power of healing. They often worked with herbs and plants and practiced through manipulation, laying on of the hands, invoking the spirits, and chanting. Throughout the Bible and Eastern literature there are references to this kind of healing. Today, unfortunately, many doctors have lost the feeling of a link between themselves and a greater power. Years of highly technical training and the reliance on drugs, surgery, and medical machinery have all contributed to this break in the chain. Western medicine is practiced in the Orient but the traditional forms of Oriental medicine, known as *kampo,* are not neglected. Kampo combines the therapies of Acupuncture, Shiatsu, *Moxa* (heat treatment of tsubos), and *Anma* (rubdown or massage) with a variety of herb-bark-root medicines, and is very much in use today.

Perhaps the reason Shiatsu and other Oriental methods are now gaining recognition in the United States is that Americans long for a personal system of healing to fill the gaps created by the highly impersonal and technical methods of modern medicine. The success of the Shiatsu pressure method depends not only on the skill with which the practitioner can use his hands, but on the psychic flow of communication between himself and his patient. This is why I call Shiatsu "touch communication." Through Shiatsu one learns to understand the patient in more than just a physical way. The Orientals tell a story of a daughter-in-law who went to a Chinese herbalist for a poison to kill her mother-in-law, who had been abnormally cruel to her. The doctor gave her tea and told her to give Shiatsu along with the tea for the duration of three months. He said the poison would work most effectively with manipulation and that death would appear to be due to natural causes. The daughter-in-law did as she was instructed. However, at the end of two and a half months she began to regret her desire to kill her mother-in-law, whom she had come to know and understand through giving her Shiatsu; at the same time, her mother-in-law started to love her because of Shiatsu. Finally, she ran back to the wise old doctor to ask for an antidote for the poison. He then told her the tea was not really poison, only flower water.

Eastern and Western Medicine

In Western medicine the area in which the patient suffers symptoms is treated. For example, if you suffer from severe headaches, the doctor will prescribe something exclusively for this area, like aspirin or depressant drugs, just to kill the pain. If you have an eye problem, you go to a doctor who knows only about eye problems, gives you glasses or a prescription, and sometimes even operates to remove the area of pain or infection. You take stomach pills for your stomach, laxatives for constipation, sleeping pills for insomnia. Western medicine divides the human anatomy into categories and regards each diseased or malfunctioning part as separate from the whole.

In the Orient we believe you are built in one piece, that it is impossible to isolate a part without considering what effect it will have on the whole. We do not concentrate on the illness, but on the entire body. We do not label disease, because all diseases come from the same source—an imbalance of energy flow throughout the body. In the East, if you have a cold, the doctor will give you Shiatsu to increase your ability to produce the energy you need to fight the cold. To the Westerner this may seem unscientific, a form of magic or mystery, but on the contrary, it is very practical and specific. We believe that if one keeps a healthy balance of energy in the body, it will fight off almost any infection. If we develop self-healing power through proper eating, breathing, and exercise, we can prevent the development of disease and disability. If, on the other hand, you lack this basic self-healing power, no amount of medicine or surgery will cure you. Shiatsu and other forms of Oriental medicine help re-establish a disrupted balance of energy, but it is the body itself that basically cures the disease. Thus, when a certain Dr. Wada performed a heart-transplant operation he was sued by a group of Japanese Eastern medicine doctors, because with their background in the subtle techniques of Acupuncture, Moxa, and Shiatsu they viewed his action as a terrible insult to the human body. They saw Dr. Wada as a representative of the most negative aspects of Western medicine—treating the human body as an automobile with interchangeable parts. Although Oriental medicine has accepted much from the West, this type of operation is still an outrage—totally counter to traditional Eastern philosophy. The only time we treat an isolated area of the body is in cases of external injury to the area. For example, if you fall and pull a muscle in your lower back and the next day feel pain in the same area, there is a mechanical reason for the backache, not one involving the body's total energy flow.

Another example of the inevitable conflict between Eastern and Western medicine occurred when General MacArthur banned Oriental medicine, such as Acupuncture, Moxa, and Shiatsu, in occupied Japan after World War II. These techniques, which MacArthur believed unscientific, and therefore useless, were being practiced by some blind people, who have highly sensitive fingers and the ability to see beyond sight. As a result, all the blind therapists lost their jobs and some committed suicide. The Japanese Blind Association sent an emergency message to Helen Keller asking her help. She wrote to President Harry Truman, who in turn put pressure on General MacArthur to change the law. Blind Shiatsu and

Acupuncture practitioners in Japan still love the memory of Helen Keller. In Tokyo, there is a Shiatsu and Acupuncture school mainly for the blind, named The Helen Keller Institute.

In Japanese my name, *Ohashi*, means "big bridge." Even in this modern, well-informed world we still need bridges between the East and the West so we can learn from each other. This is my purpose in teaching Shiatsu in America.

2. Finding the Tsubo

The fourteen major channels of energy that run through the body are called meridian lines. Each one is named for the organ or function connected to its energy flow. The meridian lines are divided into positive and negative forces—or Yang and Yin. The Yang lines begin at the top of the head, face, and fingertips and descend toward the earth or to the center of the human body. The Yin lines start from the toes and the center of the body and ascend upward toward the head and the fingertips. Stand with your feet turned out (as in a ballet first position) and your arms raised above your head (see Fig. 2–1 and Fig. 2–2). In this posture the Yin side of your body is the front and the Yang side is the back. There are six Yang meridians, three in the arms and three in the legs; six Yin meridians, three in the arms and three in the legs; and two vessel lines that run on the ventral and dorsal sides of the body. The same meridians are located on both the left and right halves of the body. It is important to know if a meridian is Yin or Yang in order to know which way the energy is flowing, so when giving Shiatsu you can work with the energy flow or against it, depending on whether you want to increase or decrease the energy level of a patient (see chapter 3, Shiatsu Technique).

The six Yang meridians are Large Intestine, Stomach, Small Intestine, Bladder, Triple Heater, and Gall Bladder. The six Yin meridians are Lung, Spleen, Kidney, Heart, Heart Constrictor, and Liver. There is, of course, no such organ in the human body as the "Heart constrictor"; this term is used to describe the function of circulation. "Triple Heater" describes the system that produces and delivers heat to all parts of the body. "Spleen" is an Oriental term for "pancreas." The Governing Vessel Meridian (Yang) and the Conception Vessel Meridian (Yin) control the energy flow in all the meridian lines and correlate their activities. All the meridian lines are most active at different times of the day, and, ideally, the tsubos along them should be pressed during that period for maximum benefit to the patient. This, however, is a bit impractical as it can mean rising at three A.M., for example, for Shiatsu treatments on the Lung Meridian.

Once you become aware of these energy channels and the ways in which they connect the different limbs, organs, and muscles of the body, your entire concept of health will change. You will begin to see the body as a kind of network of highways, with all the places in it connected di-

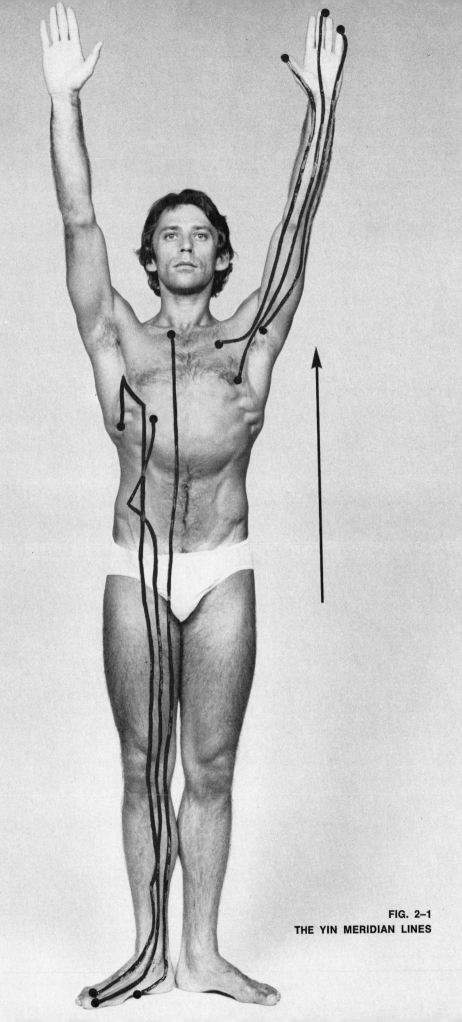

FIG. 2–1
THE YIN MERIDIAN LINES

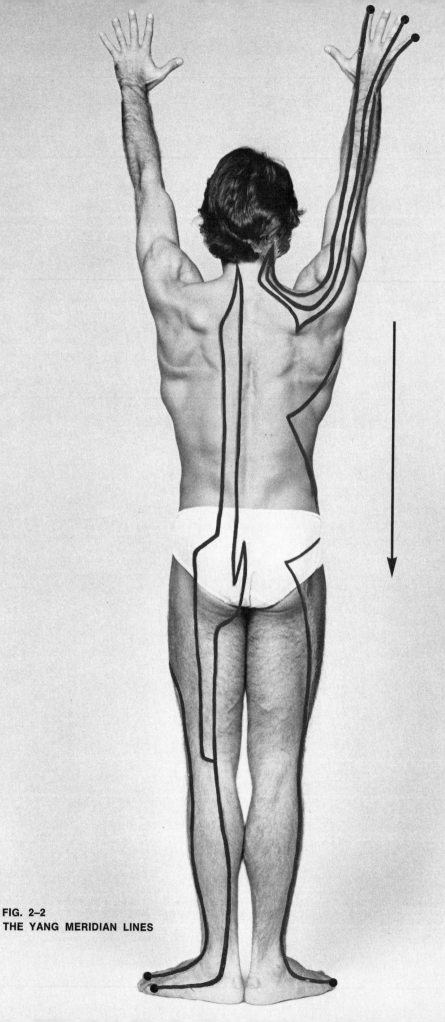

FIG. 2–2
THE YANG MERIDIAN LINES

rectly to each other. Stiffness and pain in a particular part of the body will no longer seem an isolated phenomenon, but a signal that other places along the meridian line are aching too.

We both diagnose and treat ailments in Shiatsu by stimulating pressure-sensitive points (tsubos) along the meridian lines in various ways. We can press the tsubos with the fingers, as we do in Shiatsu, stimulate them with needles (Acupuncture), and also with heat in the treatment called Moxa, where a tiny piece of an herb called mugwort is burned on the tsubo. We can also stimulate the tsubos with suction, which we create by burning something in an airtight glass cup which is placed over the tsubo in what we call "cupping technique." These different methods exert either positive or negative stimuli on the tsubo and affect them in different ways. Oddly enough, different types of stimulation applied to the same tsubo have different effects on the same ailments. For example, Governing Vessel #20 on top of the head can be treated with Shiatsu, Acupuncture, and Moxa to relieve headache and hemorrhoids, but the Moxa stimulus is more effective for hemorrhoids than the other two.

The greatest challenge to the beginning student of Shiatsu is, of course, learning to find the many tsubos on the meridian lines and to press them in a way that gives maximum benefit to the patient. In general, you know and your patient knows when you have found the tsubo, as it is an experience quite unlike any other. The tsubo is usually a highly sensitive area which often seems to be the size and shape of a fingertip. I like to tell the students in my school, "The tsubos are waiting for you." They seem virtually to spring to meet your fingertips, like a negative electric charge uniting with a positive. The tsubos are normally sensitive, but hyper-sensitivity in a tsubo is a signal to the Shiatsu practitioner that ki-energy has stagnated in that part of the body and the rest of the meridian and its associated organs have been cut off the supply line. Hypersensitivity may mean pain, but not always; extreme stiffness or a highly ticklish feeling in the tsubo may also indicate a problem. When even a light touch produces tremendous pain or hypersensitivity in a tsubo you can be sure there is trouble somewhere in the body. Some tsubo can even tell you precisely what the problem is. For example, if you have pain in Lung #6, you may possibly have hemorrhoids; in Gall Bladder #39, gallstones; in Stomach #34, stomach cramps; and in Large Intestine #4, constipation. On the ventral side of the body we have *Bo*, or Alarm Points, and on the back, *Yu*, or Associated Points, which are connected to different organs in the body and are painful to the touch when those organs are malfunctioning. Nobody likes pain, but without pain, a signal that something is destroying our bodies and that energy flow is stagnated, we would be unable to protect ourselves from outer invasion or inner destruction. One of the reasons a disease like cancer is so dangerous is that it gives us no sensation of pain until it has reached a stage where it is almost impossible to cure. Once you know the tsubos and what pain in them signifies, you have an additional way to protect your health and perceive it in danger. On the other hand, certain tsubos *must* be painful when they are pressed. If they are not, this is also an indication that something is wrong. For example, Small Intestine #11, or *Ten So*, should be painful when pressure is applied because a nerve in the shoulder blade is being pressed.

15

Of the 361 tsubos along the meridian lines we have found that from sixty to one hundred are most effective in Shiatsu. Why, you may ask, is a particular tsubo on a meridian line more effective to treat than any other tsubo on the same meridian? Although all the tsubos on a single meridian are connected to the same areas of the body, ki-energy has a greater tendency to stagnate in some tsubos than in others. Therefore, in the following pages I list and describe only the most important tsubos.

On pages 17–22 you will find reproduced the chart used in my New York school, Shiatsu Education Center of America, Non-Profit Educational Organization, P.O. Box 1001, New York, New York 10019 (Figs. 2–3, 2–4, 2–5, and 2–6). The chart shows all the meridian lines and important tsubos on the face, front, back, and sides of the body; by studying it you will learn how the tsubos and meridian lines are related to each other and to the total skeletal and muscular structure of the body. The chart also provides anatomical locations of the important tsubos, descriptions of the best techniques for pressing them, and lists the ailments they are used to treat. On the following pages I will take each meridian line separately, trace its progress through the body, and give the pressing techniques and ailments to treat. In addition, I will give you my special secrets or "gimmicks" for finding the points on your own or someone else's body in addition to the location of the points. These "gimmicks" will be more useful to the layman in finding tsubos than a lot of technical anatomical information. Since the proportions of each human body are different, the tsubos may appear to be in different places on a tall person than they are on a short person. That is why many of my "tsubo-finding" techniques require you to use the patient's *own* fingers on his own body to locate the tsubos; the proportions of his fingers correspond to the proportions of other parts of his body. In this book, then, you have two ways to approach your study of the tsubos: (1) using the chart to find each tsubo in relationship to all the other tsubos and meridian lines; and (2) my special finding techniques as well as the photographic illustrations of each meridian line and the tsubos on it. I have also included several tsubos not on my chart which are useful for treating ailments mentioned in chapter 11. You can locate them by checking the illustration of the individual meridian line.

The best procedure for studying the tsubos is as follows: First learn the English and/or Japanese name of the tsubo. (I prefer the Japanese names because they often give the history, purpose, and location of the tsubos, as you will see by those I have translated into English. To me, the numerical English names are merely mechanistic "telephone numbers.") Then study the location and try to find the tsubos on yourself or someone else. We have used as few anatomical terms as possible, but if names of parts of the body give you trouble consult a good anatomy text such as *Gray's Anatomy*. It is unfortunately impossible for me to define all the parts of the body in layman's terms in the limited space of this book.

In Shiatsu, there is no substitute for experience. In the end, charts can help you only if you sensitize your fingers and teach them to recognize the tsubos. You can buy an expensive Acupressure point machine to find tsubos for you, but using a machine to find tsubos defeats the most important purpose of Shiatsu—cultivating the sensitivity of the fingers and learning to know someone close to you by touching him or her.

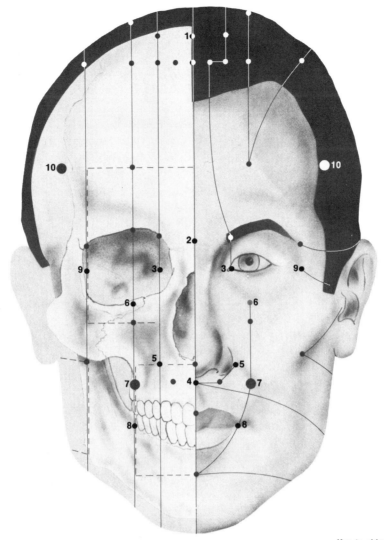

Key to abbreviations
Loc   Location of points on the figures
Tec   Technique for pressing points
For   For treatment of the ailment

FIG. 2–3 OHASHI'S CHART: FACE

上星 **1   Jo Sei (Governing Vessel #23)**
Loc: 1 inch behind the front hair line.
Tec: Press with two thumbs, hard and in, 7-10
seconds, three times.
For: Headaches and empyema (abscess in the
pleural space).

印堂 **2   In Do**
Loc: Between the eyebrows.
Tec: Press with two thumbs, hard and in, 7-10
seconds, three times.
For: Headaches and nasal obstruction.

晴明 **3   Sei Mei (Bladder #1)**
Loc: In the center of the crease within the inner
canthus of the eye. With the eye closed, the point
is 1/10 inch medial and slightly superior to the
medial canthus of the eye.
Tec: Press with one thumb or index, hard and in,
10-15 seconds, three times.
For: Poor and tired vision and red swollen eyes.

人中 **4   Nin Chu (Governing Vessel #26)**
Loc: ⅓ the distance down from the base of the
nose to the edge of the upper lip.
Tec: Press with index finger or a pointed object,
hard and in, 7-10 seconds, three times.
For: Loss of consciousness and epilepsy.

迎香 **5   Gei Ko (Large Intestine #20)**
Loc: Outside the ala nasi in the groove along the
naso-oral fold.
Tec: Press with index finger, hard and in, 10-15
seconds, three times.

For: Nasal obstruction, running nose and facial
tension.

承泣 **6   Sho Kyu (Stomach #1)**
Loc: Immediately superior to the midpoint of the
infraorbital margin and directly below the pupils
when looking straight forward.
Tec: Press with index finger, hard and in, 10-15
seconds, three times.
For: Facial pain and tension and tired vision.

巨髎 **7   Kyo Sho (Stomach #3)**
Loc: Lateral to the base of the nose and on the
line directly below the pupils when looking straight
forward.
Tec: Press with index finger, hard and in, 5-7
seconds, three times.
For: Sinus, facial pain and tension.

地倉 **8   Chi So (Stomach #4)**
Loc: Lateral to the corner of the mouth and on a
line directly below the pupils when looking straight
forward.
Tec: Press with index finger, hard and in, 5-7
seconds, three times.
For: Stomach ache, facial tension and tension.

瞳子髎 **9   Do Shi Ryo (Gall Bladder #1)**
Loc: ½ inch from outer canthus of the eye.
Tec: Press with index finger, softly and in, 10-15
seconds, three times.
For: Eye problems and headaches.

太陽 **10   Tai Yo**
Loc: One finger's width lateral to the eyebrow and
the outer canthus, in the fossa.
Tec: Press in with one thumb, gradually and hard,
7-10 seconds, three times.
For: Headaches, red swollen eyes and dizziness.

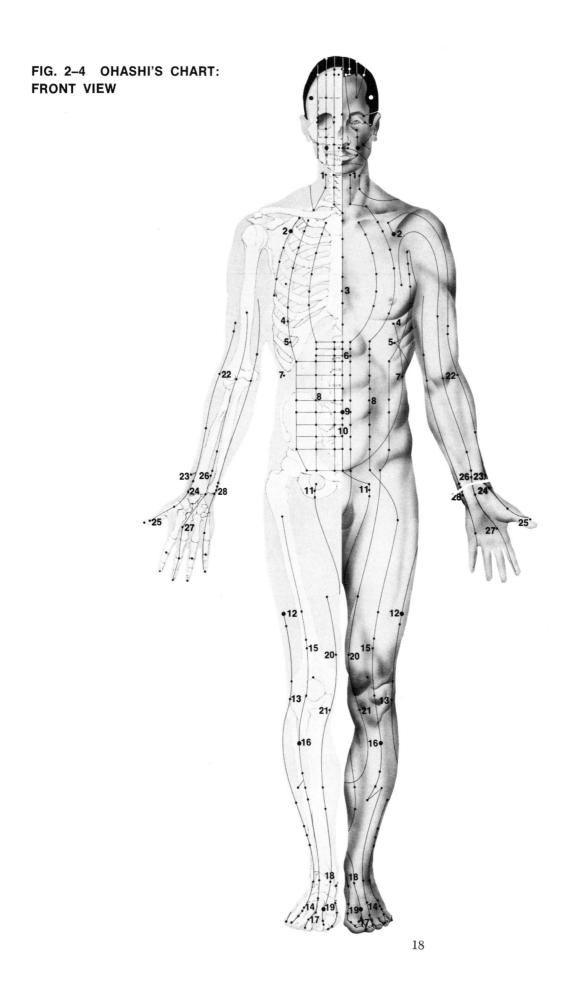

FIG. 2–4 OHASHI'S CHART: FRONT VIEW

人迎 **1 Jin Gei (Stomach #9)**
Loc: Point is 1½ inches from the middle line on the larynx, where a small pulse is felt.
Tec: Press with one thumb, softly and in, 10-15 seconds, three times.
For: High blood pressure.

中府 **2 Chu Fu (Lung #1)**
Loc: Point is located 1 inch below the middle of the clavicle.
Tec: Press with one thumb, hard and in, 7-10 seconds, three times.
For: Common cold, cough and asthma.

臍中 **3 Dan Chu (Conception Vessel #17)**
Loc: Middle of the sternum, at the level of the nipples. Level with the 4th intercostal space.
Tec: Press with two thumbs, softly and in, 10-15 seconds, three times.
For: Asthma, high blood pressure and lack of milk.

期門 **4 Ki Mon (Liver #14)**
Loc: Between the 6th and 7th rib.
Tec: Press with one thumb, softly and in, 5-10 seconds, three times.
For: Rib pains and lack of milk.

日月 **5 Jitsu Getsu (Gall Bladder #24)**
Loc: Between the 7th and 8th ribs.
Tec: Press with one thumb, hard and in, 7-10 seconds, three times.
For: Gall bladder ailments.

中脘 **6 Chu Kan (Conception Vessel #12)**
Loc: Medial abdominal line, 4 inches above the navel.
Tec: Press with the palm of the hand, down and softly, 10-15 seconds, three times.
For: Nausea, vomiting and diarrhea.

章門 **7 Shyo Mon (Liver #13)**
Loc: At the end of the rib cage.
Tec: Press with one thumb, hard and in, 7-10 seconds, three times.
For: Abdominal pain and vomiting.

天枢 **8 Ten Su (Stomach #25)**
Loc: 2 inches laterally from the navel.
Tec: Press with three fingers, gradually, in and deep, 10-15 seconds, three times.
For: Abdominal pain and diarrhea.

気海 **9 Ki Kai (Conception Vessel #6)**
Loc: 1½ inches below the navel.
Tec: Press with the palm of the hand, gradually, in and deep, 10-15 seconds, three times.
For: Stomach pains, diarrhea, wet dreams, menstrual irregularities, and constipation.

関元 **10 Kan Gen (Conception Vessel #4)**
Loc: 3 inches below the navel.
Tec: Press with the palm of the hand, gradually, in and deep, 10-15 seconds, three times.
For: Wet dreams, frigidity, impotence and menstrual irregularities.

陰廉 **11 In Ren (Liver #11)**
Loc: 2 inches down from the crease between the legs and torso.
Tec: Press with one thumb, hard and in, 5-10 seconds, three times.
For: Menstrual irregularities and frigidity.

風市 **12 Fu Shi (Gall Bladder #31)**
Loc: Lateral thigh, at the tip of the middle finger when arms are straight down.
Tec: Press with two thumbs, gradually, deep and in, 10-15 seconds, three times.
For: Circulation of the legs and tired legs.

陽陵泉 **13 Yo Ryo Sen (Gall Bladder #33)**
Loc: Just under the knee cap, on top of the fibula and on lateral leg.
Tec: Press with one thumb, hard and in, 7-10 seconds, three times.
For: Fevers and paralysis of the legs.

臨泣 **14 Rin Kyu (Gall Bladder #41)**
Loc: In the depression between the 4th and 5th metatarsus.
Tec: Press with one thumb, in and up, softly, 5-10 seconds, three times.
For: Menstrual irregularities, ringing in the ears and foot pain.

梁丘 **15 Ryo Kyu (Stomach #34)**
Loc: In the fossa 2 inches above the lower end of the femur, on the lateral side. 2 inches directly proximal to the lateral edge of the base of the patella.
Tec: Press with one thumb, hard and in, 7-10 seconds, three times.
For: Stomach pains, cramps and arthritis in the knee.

三里 **16 Ashi San Ri (Stomach #36)**
Loc: 3 inches below Stomach-35, one finger's width below the tibial tuberosity, on top of the anterior tibial muscle. It is located in the depression between the tibia and the tibialis anticus muscle.
Tec: Press with two thumbs, hard and in, 10-15 seconds, three times.
For: General well-being.

内庭 **17 Nai Tei (Stomach #44)**
Loc: Between the 2nd and 3rd toes, in the groove of the depression near the 2nd phalanges.
Tec: Press with one thumb, hard and up, 7-10 seconds, three times.
For: Toothaches and stomach aches.

中封 **18 Chu Ho (Liver #4)**
Loc: Just between the anklebone and the extensors.
Tec: Press with one thumb, hard and in, 7-10 seconds, three times.
For: Arthritis in the ankle.

太衝 **19 Tai Chu (Liver #3)**
Loc: 1½ inches up between the 1st and 2nd metatarsals.
Tec: Press with one thumb, hard and up, 7-10 seconds, three times.
For: Headaches and dizziness.

血海 **20 Ketsu Kai (Spleen #10)**
Loc: 2 inches above the patella, at the bulge of the medial vastus muscle.
Tec: Press with two thumbs, hard and in, 5-10 seconds, three times.
For: Itch, allergic eczema, hives and menstrual irregularities.

陰陵泉 **21 Yin Ryo Sen (Spleen #9)**
Loc: At the top of the tibia, on the inside of the leg.
Tec: Press with one thumb, hard and in, 7-10 seconds, three times.
For: Pain in the knee.

尺沢 **22 Shoku Taku (Lung #5)**
Loc: In the elbow fold, on the radial side of the biceps. It can be seen when the arm is slightly bent.
Tec: Press with one thumb, hard and in, 7-10 seconds, three times.
For: Cough, elbow pain and labored breathing.

列欠 **23 Retsu Kyu (Lung #7)**
Loc: On top of the radial tuberosity, 1½ inches above the wrist fold.
Tec: Press with one thumb, hard and in, 7-10 seconds, three times.
For: Common colds, headaches and Bell's palsy.

太淵 **24 Tai En (Lung #9)**
Loc: On the ventral surface of the wrist, below the wrist fold, in between the radial artery and the depression at the lateral side of the radius, where a small pulse can be felt.
Tec: Press with one thumb, hard and in, 7-10 seconds, three times.
For: Labored breathing, cough, and pharyngitis.

少商 **25 Shou Shu (Lung #11)**
Loc: On the radial side of the thumb, 1/10 inch to the side from the base of the nail.
Tec: Press with a pointed object, hard and in, 7-10 seconds, three times.
For: Sore throat, cough, pharyngitis, hand spasms and tired arms.

内関 **26 Nai Kan (Heart Constrictor #6)**
Loc: 2 inches above the wrist fold, in between the tendon longus volaris and the tendon flexor carpi radialis.
Tec: Press with one thumb, hard and in, 7-10 seconds, three times.
For: Nausea, vomiting, insomnia and palpitations.

労宮 **27 Ro Kyu (Heart Constrictor #8)**
Loc: On the palm, 1 inch from the 3rd metacarpo-phalangeal joint, between the 2nd and 3rd metacarpals. It can also be located at the point where the tip of the completely flexed middle finger touches the most distal major palmar crease.
Tec: Press with one thumb, hard and in, 10-15 seconds, three times.
For: Exhaustion.

神門 **28 Shin Mon (Heart #7)**
Loc: In the joint between the plisiform and the ulna. In the fossa of the radial side of the musculus flexor carpi ulnaris.
Tec: Press with one thumb, hard and in, 7-10 seconds, three times.
For: Irritability and insomnia.

Key to abbreviations
Loc Location of points on the figures
Tec Technique for pressing points
For For treatment of the ailment

19

**FIG. 2–5
OHASHI'S CHART:
BACK VIEW**

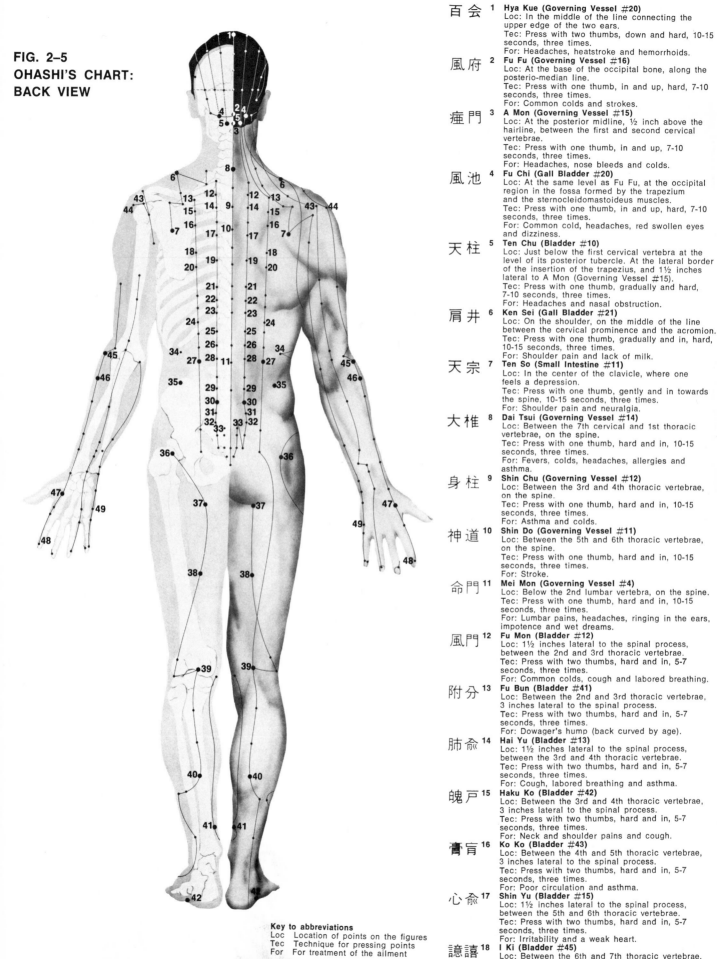

Key to abbreviations
Loc Location of points on the figures
Tec Technique for pressing points
For For treatment of the ailment

百会 **1 Hya Kue (Governing Vessel #20)**
Loc: In the middle of the line connecting the upper edge of the two ears.
Tec: Press with two thumbs, down and hard, 10-15 seconds, three times.
For: Headaches, heatstroke and hemorrhoids.

風府 **2 Fu Fu (Governing Vessel #16)**
Loc: At the base of the occipital bone, along the posterio-median line.
Tec: Press with one thumb, in and up, hard, 7-10 seconds, three times.
For: Common colds and strokes.

瘂門 **3 A Mon (Governing Vessel #15)**
Loc: At the posterior midline, ½ inch above the hairline, between the first and second cervical vertebrae.
Tec: Press with one thumb, in and up, 7-10 seconds, three times.
For: Headaches, nose bleeds and colds.

風池 **4 Fu Chi (Gall Bladder #20)**
Loc: At the same level as Fu Fu, at the occipital region in the fossa formed by the trapezium and the sternocleidomastoideus muscles.
Tec: Press with one thumb, in and up, hard, 7-10 seconds, three times.
For: Common cold, headaches, red swollen eyes and dizziness.

天柱 **5 Ten Chu (Bladder #10)**
Loc: Just below the first cervical vertebra at the level of its posterior tubercle. At the lateral border of the insertion of the trapezius, and 1½ inches lateral to A Mon (Governing Vessel #15).
Tec: Press with one thumb, gradually and hard, 7-10 seconds, three times.
For: Headaches and nasal obstruction.

肩井 **6 Ken Sei (Gall Bladder #21)**
Loc: On the shoulder, on the middle of the line between the cervical prominence and the acromion.
Tec: Press with one thumb, gradually and in, hard, 10-15 seconds, three times.
For: Shoulder pain and lack of milk.

天宗 **7 Ten So (Small Intestine #11)**
Loc: In the center of the clavicle, where one feels a depression.
Tec: Press with one thumb, gently and in towards the spine, 10-15 seconds, three times.
For: Shoulder pain and neuralgia.

大椎 **8 Dai Tsui (Governing Vessel #14)**
Loc: Between the 7th cervical and 1st thoracic vertebrae, on the spine.
Tec: Press with one thumb, hard and in, 10-15 seconds, three times.
For: Fevers, colds, headaches, allergies and asthma.

身柱 **9 Shin Chu (Governing Vessel #12)**
Loc: Between the 3rd and 4th thoracic vertebrae, on the spine.
Tec: Press with one thumb, hard and in, 10-15 seconds, three times.
For: Asthma and colds.

神道 **10 Shin Do (Governing Vessel #11)**
Loc: Between the 5th and 6th thoracic vertebrae, on the spine.
Tec: Press with one thumb, hard and in, 10-15 seconds, three times.
For: Stroke.

命門 **11 Mei Mon (Governing Vessel #4)**
Loc: Below the 2nd lumbar vertebra, on the spine.
Tec: Press with one thumb, hard and in, 10-15 seconds, three times.
For: Lumbar pains, headaches, ringing in the ears, impotence and wet dreams.

風門 **12 Fu Mon (Bladder #12)**
Loc: 1½ inches lateral to the spinal process, between the 2nd and 3rd thoracic vertebrae.
Tec: Press with two thumbs, hard and in, 5-7 seconds, three times.
For: Common colds, cough and labored breathing.

附分 **13 Fu Bun (Bladder #41)**
Loc: Between the 2nd and 3rd thoracic vertebrae, 3 inches lateral to the spinal process.
Tec: Press with two thumbs, hard and in, 5-7 seconds, three times.
For: Dowager's hump (back curved by age).

肺俞 **14 Hai Yu (Bladder #13)**
Loc: 1½ inches lateral to the spinal process, between the 3rd and 4th thoracic vertebrae.
Tec: Press with two thumbs, hard and in, 5-7 seconds, three times.
For: Cough, labored breathing and asthma.

魄戸 **15 Haku Ko (Bladder #42)**
Loc: Between the 3rd and 4th thoracic vertebrae, 3 inches lateral to the spinal process.
Tec: Press with two thumbs, hard and in, 5-7 seconds, three times.
For: Neck and shoulder pains and cough.

膏肓 **16 Ko Ko (Bladder #43)**
Loc: Between the 4th and 5th thoracic vertebrae, 3 inches lateral to the spinal process.
Tec: Press with two thumbs, hard and in, 5-7 seconds, three times.
For: Poor circulation and asthma.

心俞 **17 Shin Yu (Bladder #15)**
Loc: 1½ inches lateral to the spinal process, between the 5th and 6th thoracic vertebrae.
Tec: Press with two thumbs, hard and in, 5-7 seconds, three times.
For: Irritability and a weak heart.

譩譆 **18 I Ki (Bladder #45)**
Loc: Between the 6th and 7th thoracic vertebrae, 3 inches lateral to the spinal process.

膈俞 19 **Kaku Yu (Bladder #17)**
Loc: Between the 7th and 8th thoracic vertebrae, 1½ inches lateral to the spinal process.
Tec: Press with two thumbs, hard and in, 5-7 seconds, three times.
For: Pains along the ribs, stomach ache and hiccups.

膈関 20 **Kaku Kan (Bladder #46)**
Loc: Between the 7th and 8th thoracic vertebrae, 3 inches lateral to the spinal process.
Tec: Press with two thumbs, hard and in, 5-7 seconds, three times.
For: Nausea, vomiting and hiccups.

肝俞 21 **Kan Yu (Bladder #18)**
Loc: Between the 9th and 10th thoracic vertebrae, 1½ inches lateral to the spinal process.
Tec: Press with two thumbs, hard and in, 5-7 seconds, three times.
For: Pains along the ribs, dizziness, seasickness and liver locus.

胆俞 22 **Tan Yu (Bladder #19)**
Loc: Between the 10th and 11th thoracic vertebrae, 1½ inches lateral to the spinal process.
Tec: Press with two thumbs, hard and in, 5-7 seconds, three times.
For: Pains along the ribs, dry mouth and gall bladder locus.

脾俞 23 **Hi Yu (Bladder #20)**
Loc: Between the 11th and 12th thoracic vertebrae, 1½ inches lateral to the spinal process.
Tec: Press with two thumbs, hard and in, 5-7 seconds, three times.
For: Diabetes, loss of appetite and spleen locus.

意舎 24 **I Sha (Bladder #49)**
Loc: Between the 11th and 12th thoracic vertebrae, three inches lateral to the spinal process.
Tec: Press with two thumbs, hard and in, 5-7 seconds, three times.
For: Diarrhea, stomach ache and nervous trouble.

胃俞 25 **I Yu (Bladder #21)**
Loc: Between the 12th thoracic and 1st lumbar vetebrae, 1½ inches lateral to the spinal process.
Tec: Press with two thumbs, hard and in, 5-7 seconds, three times.
For: Stomach ache and stomach locus.

三焦俞 26 **San Shyo Yu (Bladder #22)**
Loc: Between the 1st and 2nd lumbar vertebrae, 1½ inches lateral to the spinal process.
Tec: Press with two thumbs, hard and in, 5-7 seconds, three times.
For: Diarrhea, exhaustion, lower-back ache and "triple heater" locus.

志室 27 **Shi Shitsu (Bladder #52)**
Loc: Between the 2nd and 3rd lumbar vertebrae, 3 inches lateral to the spinal process.
Tec: Press with two thumbs, hard and in, towards the spine, 5-7 seconds, three times.
For: Lower backache, exhaustion and sexual strength.

腎俞 28 **Jin Yu (Bladder #23)**
Loc: Between the 2nd and 3rd lumbar vertebrae, 1½ inches lateral to the spinal process.
Tec: Press with two thumbs, hard and in, 5-7 seconds, three times.
For: Weakness and kidney locus.

大腸俞 29 **Dai Chyo Yu (Bladder #25)**
Loc: At the level of the transtubercular plain, 1½ inches lateral to the spinal process of the 4th lumbar vertebra.
Tec: Press with two thumbs, hard and in, 5-7 seconds, three times.
For: Diarrhea, constipation and large intestine locus.

関元俞 30 **Kan Gen Yu (Bladder #26)**
Loc: Between the 5th lumbar vertebra and the pelvic bone, 1½ inches lateral to the spinal process.
Tec: Press with two thumbs, hard and in, 5-7 seconds, three times.
For: Lower-back ache, digestion and sexual strength.

小腸俞 31 **Sho Cho Yu (Bladder #27)**
Loc: In the fossa at the level of the 1st sacral foramen and 1½ inches lateral to the central line of the body.
Tec: Press with two thumbs, hard and in, 5-7 seconds, three times.
For: Lower-back ache, hip pain and small intestine locus.

膀胱俞 32 **Bo Ko Yu (Bladder #28)**
Loc: In the fossa at the level of the 2nd sacral foramen and 1½ inches lateral to the central line of the body.
Tec: Press with two thumbs, hard and in, 5-7 seconds, three times.
For: Bed-wetting and bladder locus.

次髎 33 **Gi Ryo (Bladder #32)**
Loc: In the 2nd foramen.
Tec: Press with two thumbs, hard and in, 5-7 seconds, three times.
For: Bed-wetting and menstrual irregularities.

京門 34 **Kei Mon (Gall Bladder #25)**
Loc: Below 12th rib.
Tec: Press with one thumb, hard and in, 7-10 seconds, three times.
For: Stomach ache, digestion and vomiting.

転子 35 **Ten Shi**
Loc: About 3 inches lateral to the hip bone.

Tec: Press toward the sacrum with two thumbs, hard and in, 10-15 seconds, three times.
For: Lower-back ache, sexual strength and digestion.

環跳 36 **Kan Chyo (Gall Bladder #30)**
Loc: At ⅓ distance from the great trochanter to the last hole of the sacrum.
Tec: Press with two thumbs, hard and in, 10-15 seconds, three times.
For: Sciatica and lower-back ache.

承扶 37 **Sho Fu (Bladder #36)**
Loc: At the midline on the posterior surface of the thigh, and at the level of the gluteal fold.
Tec: Press with two thumbs, hard and up, 10-15 seconds, three times.
For: Sciatica and lower-back ache.

殷門 38 **I Mon (Bladder #37)**
Loc: At the midline of the posterior surface of the thigh, and 6 inches from the gluteal fold, or halfway between Bladder #36, Sho-Fu, and Bladder #40, I Chu.
Tec: Press with two thumbs, hard and in, and up, 10-15 seconds, three times.
For: Sciatica and tired legs.

委中 39 **I Chu (Bladder #40)**
Loc: At the center of the polipteal fossa.
Tec: Press with two thumbs, soft and in, 7-10 seconds, three times.
For: Sciatica, lower-back ache and calf spasms.

承山 40 **Sho Zan (Bladder #57)**
Loc: In the gastrocnemius muscles. Stretch the lower leg and a cross depression appears, in the gastrocnemius.
Tec: Press with one thumb, softly and in, 10-15 seconds, three times.
For: Sciatica, spasms of the gastrocnemius and tired legs.

三陰交 41 **San Yin Ko (Spleen #6)**
Loc: 3 inches above the medial malleolus, along the posterior ridge of the tibia.
Tec: Press with two thumbs, hard and in, toward the bone, 7-10 seconds, three times.
For: Traumatic pain in the ankles, overweight, digestive problems, insomnia and menstrual irregularities.

湧泉 42 **Yu Sen (Kidney #1)**
Loc: Located on the sole of the foot at ⅓ the distance from the tip of the middle toe, to the heel, and on the crease formed when the toes are flexed.
Tec: Press with two thumbs, hard and in, 10-15 seconds, three times.
For: Epilepsy, dizziness and menstrual irregularities.

肩髎 43 **Ken Ryo (Triple Heater #14)**
Loc: On the dorsal surface of the shoulder at the bottom of the crease formed below the acromion where the arm is lifted.
Tec: Press with two thumbs, hard and in, 10-15 seconds, three times.
For: Shoulder joint pains.

肩髃 44 **Ken Gu (Large Intestine #15)**
Loc: Between the acromion and the greater tubercle of the humerus and in the middle of the upper deltoid. For the identification of this locus, when the patient's arm is abducted to a horizontal position, two depressions will appear below the acromion and the clavicle; the smaller depression immediately anterior to the distal tip of the acromion is the point.
Tec: Press with two thumbs, hard and in, 10-15 seconds, three times.
For: Shoulder joint pains.

曲池 45 **Kyoku Chi (Large Intestine #11)**
Loc: At the depression of the end of the fold which appears when the elbow is bent 90 degrees and abducted to a horizontal position.
Tec: Press with one thumb, hard, towards elbow, 10-15 seconds, three times.
For: Diarrhea, headache, fever and arm pains.

三里 46 **Te San Ri (Large Intestine #10)**
Loc: 1½ inches from Large Intestine-11, Kyoku Chi.
Tec: Press with one thumb, hard and in, 7-10 seconds, three times.
For: General well-being.

合谷 47 **Go Koku (Large Intestine #4)**
Loc: Between the 1st and 2nd metacarpi. Near the radial side of the middle of the 2nd metacarpus. When fingers are held together, the locus is found below the fleshy mound that forms between the base of the thumb and the index finger. With the index and thumb held at 90 degrees to each other, the therapist should catch webbing between the thumb and index finger with the 1st phalange of the thumb to locate the point at the tip of his thumb.
Tec: Press with one thumb, hard, towards index finger, 10-15 seconds, three times.
For: Diarrhea, rashes, facial tension and toothaches.

商陽 48 **Sho Yo (Large Intestine #1)**
Loc: On the radial side of the index finger, 1/10 inch to the side of the base of the nail.
Tec: Press with a pointed object, hard and in, 5-7 seconds, three times.
For: Fevers and diarrhea.

後谿 49 **Go Kei (Small Intestine #3)**
Loc: Locus is on the fold that appears when the hand is making a fist, behind the 5th finger at the cubital edge of the hand.
Tec: Press with thumb or a pointed object, hard and in, 7-10 seconds, three times.
For: Numbness and paralysis of the fingers and headaches.

FIG. 2–6 OHASHI'S CHART: SIDE VIEW

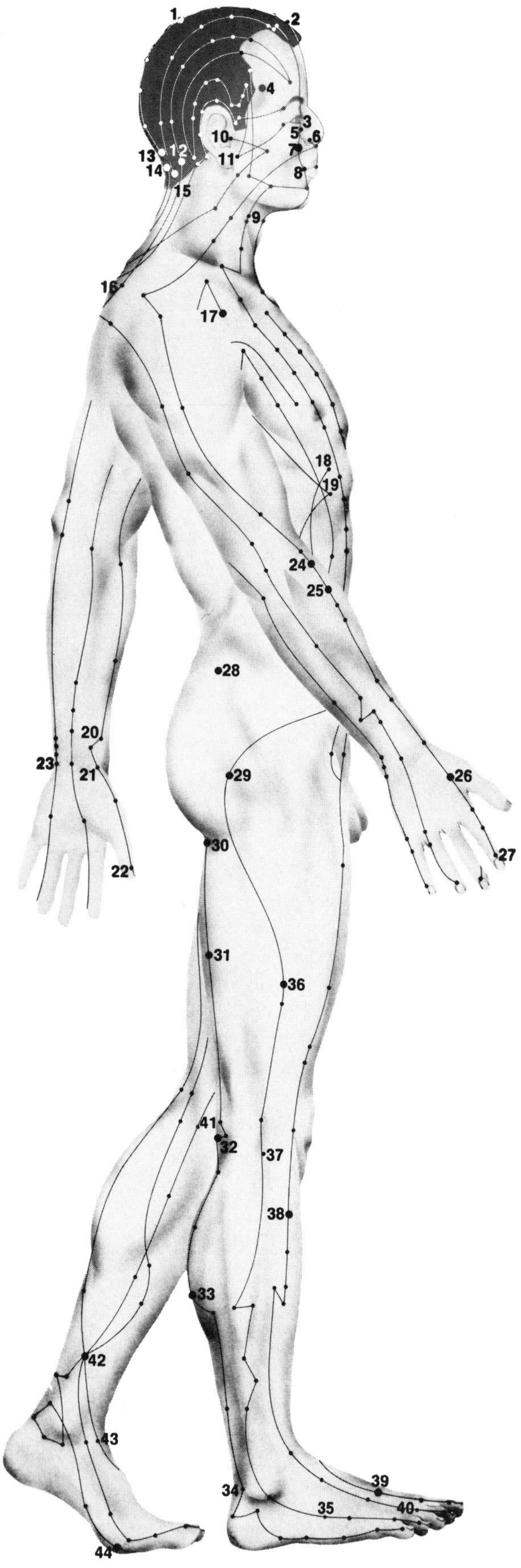

百会 **1 Hya Kue (Governing Vessel #20)**
See Back 1

上星 **2 Jo Sei (Governing Vessel #23)**
See Face 1

晴明 **3 Sei Mei (Bladder #1)**
See Face 3

太陽 **4 Tai Yo**
See Face 10

承泣 **5 Sho Kyu (Stomach #1)**
See Face 6

迎香 **6 Gei Ko (Large Intestine #20)**
See Face 5

巨髎 **7 Kyo Sho (Stomach #3)**
See Face 7

地倉 **8 Chi So (Stomach #4)**
See Face 8

人迎 **9 Jin Gei (Stomach #9)**
See Front 1

聴宮 **10 Chyo Ku (Small Intestine #19)**
Loc: In front of the tragus at the depression made when the mouth is slightly open.
Tec: Press with index finger, hard and in, 7–10 seconds, three times.
For: Ringing in the ears.

聴会 **11 Cho E (Gall Bladder #2)**
Loc: Just below Small Intestine-19, Chyo Ku.
Tec: Press with index finger, hard and in, 7–10 seconds, three times.
For: Ringing in the ears.

風池 **12 Fu Chi (Gall Bladder #20)**
See Back 4

風府 **13 Fu Fu (Governing Vessel #16)**
See Back 2

瘂門 **14 A Mon (Governing Vessel #15)**
See Back 3

天柱 **15 Ten Chu (Bladder #10)**
See Back 5

肩髃 **16 Ken Gu (Large Intestine #15)**
See Back 44

中府 **17 Chu Fu (Lung #1)**
See Front 2

期門 **18 Ki Mon (Liver #14)**
See Front 4

日月 **19 Jitsu Getsu (Gall Bladder #24)**
See Front 5

列欠 **20 Rei Ketsu (Lung #7)**
See Front 23

太淵 **21 Tai En (Lung #9)**
See Front 24

少商 **22 Shou Sho (Lung #11)**
See Front 25

神門 **23 Shin Mon (Heart #7)**
See Front 28

曲池 **24 Kyoku Chi (Large Intestine #11)**
See Back 45

三里 **25 Te San Ri (Large Intestine #10)**
See Back 46

合谷 **26 Go Koku (Large Intestine #4)**
See Back 47

商陽 **27 Sho Yo (Large Intestine #1)**
See Back 48

轉子 **28 Ten Shi**
See Back 35

環跳 **29 Kan Chyo (Gall Bladder #30)**
See Back 36

承扶 **30 Sho Fu (Bladder #36)**
See Back 37

殷門 **31 I Mon (Bladder #37)**
See Back 38

委中 **32 I Chu (Bladder #40)**
See Back 39

承山 **33 Shyo Zan (Bladder #57)**
See Back 40

崑崙 **34 Kon Ron (Bladder #60)**
Loc: Between the external malleolus and the Achilles tendon.
Tec: Press with one thumb, hard and in, 7–10 seconds, three times.
For: Sciatica, dizziness and epilepsy.

臨泣 **35 Rin Kyu (Gall Bladder #40)**
See Front 14

風市 **36 Fu Shi (Gall Bladder #31)**
See Front 12

陽陵泉 **37 Yo Ryo Sen (Gall Bladder #33)**
See Front 13

三里 **38 Ashi San Ri (Stomach #36)**
See Front 16

太衝 **39 Tai Chu (Liver #3)**
See Front 19

内庭 **40 Nai Tei (Stomach #44)**
See Front 17

陰陵泉 **41 In Ryo Sen (Spleen #9)**
See Front 21

三陰交 **42 San Yin Ko (Spleen #6)**
See Back 41

中封 **43 Chu Fu (Liver #4)**
See Front 18

湧泉 **44 Yu Sen (Kidney #1)**
See Back 42

Key to abbreviations
Loc Location of points on the figures
Tec Technique for pressing points
For For treatment of the ailment

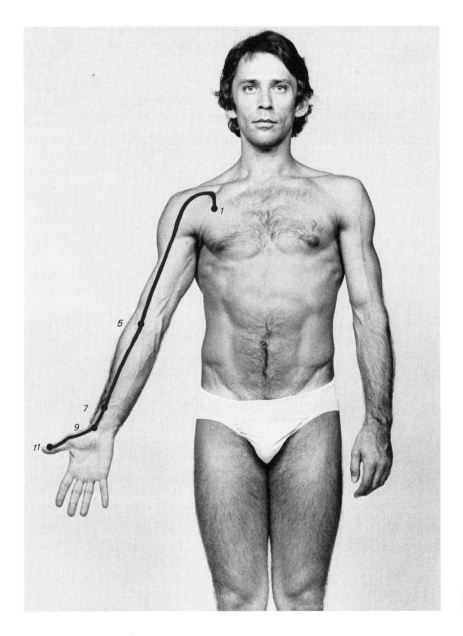

FIG. 2-7
LUNG MERIDIAN

Major Tsubos on the Meridian Lines

1. LUNG MERIDIAN (Yin) Fig. 2-7

Lung #1 Chu Fu ("center of gathering") Fig. 2-8

Location: Measure two inches from the nipple (in the direction of the arm). Count up three ribs. The point is between the first and second ribs from the top, one inch below the middle of the clavicle.

Technique: Press with one thumb for 7–10 seconds.

For: Common cold, cough, asthma.

Lung #5 Shoku Taku ("in the groove")

Location: Make a fist; bend the elbow. Lung #5 is on the outside of the tendon, in the fold of the elbow.

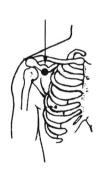

FIG. 2-8
LOCATION OF LUNG #1

23

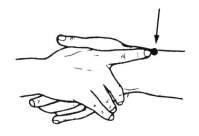

FIG. 2-9
HOW TO FIND LUNG #7

Technique: Press back and inward with one thumb for 7-10 seconds, three times.

For: Cough, elbow pain, painful breathing, stiffness, fever associated with lung problems.

Lung #7   Retsu Ketsu* Fig. 2-9

Location: Open the patient's thumb and index finger and slide his other hand in the space between them. His index finger should meet the point on the other wrist. Lung #7 is one and a half inches above the wrist fold.

Technique: Press hard and inward with one thumb for 7-10 seconds, three times.

For: Congestion, headaches, colds, Bell's palsy.

Lung #9   Tai En ("great stagnation")

Location: Make a fist and bend at the wrist. Lung #9 is in the indentation on the first fold on the thumb side of the wrist, where a small pulse can be felt.

Technique: Press hard and inward with one thumb for 7-10 seconds, three times.

For: Reviving an unconscious person (stimulate by pressing the point and rubbing hand), painful breathing, cough, pharyngitis.

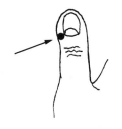

FIG. 2-10
LOCATION OF LUNG #11

Lung #11   Shou Shu ("young merchant")

Location: On outside of the thumb, one-tenth of an inch to the side from the base of the nail.

How to find: See Fig. 2-10.

Technique: Press hard and inward with a sharp pointed object, like a toothpick, for 7-10 seconds, three times.

For: Sore throat, cough, painful breathing.

2. LARGE INTESTINE MERIDIAN (Yang) Fig. 2-11

Large Intestine #1   Sho Yo ("Yang merchant")

Location: On thumb side of index finger, one-tenth of an inch to the side of base of the nail.

Technique: Press hard with a sharp pointed object for 7-10 seconds, three times.

For: Fever, diarrhea.

Large Intestine #4   Go Koku ("meeting mountains")

Location: Midway between the two bones of thumb and index finger.

How to find: Take the patient's thumb and place it in the space between his thumb and index finger on the other hand (Fig. 2-12). Bend his thumb. The tip will touch Large Intestine #4.

Technique: Press hard with one thumb toward the index finger for 10-15 seconds, three times.

For: Diarrhea, rash, pain of toothache, facial tension, important for general health.

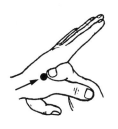

FIG. 2-12
FINDING LARGE
INTESTINE #4

* This tsubo and certain other tsubos to follow are untranslatable.

24

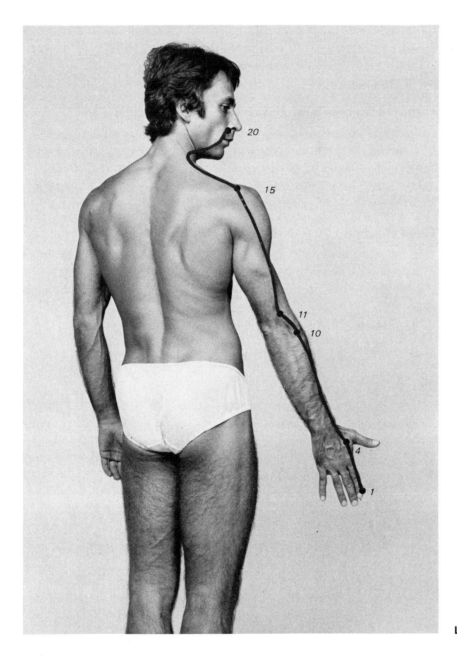

FIG. 2–11
LARGE INTESTINE MERIDIAN

Large Intestine #10   Te San Ri ("three miles")

Location: One and a half inches below depression of end of fold which appears when elbow is bent 90 degrees.

How to find: Measure three fingers' width down the forearm from the tip of the elbow crease on the outside. See Large Intestine #11.

Technique: Press hard with one thumb for 10–15 seconds, three times.

For: Sore legs, pain and fatigue in the arms, general well-being.

Large Intestine #11   Kyoku Chi
("the Lake of Energy on the corner")

Location: At the depression at the end of the fold which appears when the elbow is bent 90 degrees.

How to find: Bend the elbow. The point is at the end of the crease on the outside, halfway between Lung #5 and the top of the funny bone. It is easier to find Large Intestine #10 after you find this one.

Technique: Press hard with one thumb for 10–15 seconds, three times.

For: Any arm problem.

Large Intestine #15   Ken Gu ("corner of the shoulder")

Location: On the indentation on the outside of the shoulder bone.

How to find: Have the patient raise his bent elbow to an angle of 90 degrees from the body. The indentation will be easier to see.

Technique: Press hard with one thumb for 10–15 seconds, three times.

For: Shoulder joint pains, frozen shoulder.

Large Intestine #20   Gei Ko ("welcome smell")

Location: In the small grooves on the sides of the nose just outside the widest point of the nostrils.

Technique: Press hard and inward at a 45-degree angle with the index finger for 10–15 seconds, three times.

For: Nasal obstruction, running nose, facial tension.

3. STOMACH MERIDIAN (Yang) Fig. 2–13

Stomach #3   Kyo Sho

Location: On the line directly below the pupils when looking straight forward, parallel to the base of the nose.

How to find: See illustration of Stomach Meridian (Fig. 2–13).

Technique: Put the little finger on point first, cover with the thumb, then press up and in toward the eye.

For: Sinus, nose congestion, facial pain or paralysis, tension.

Stomach #4   Chi So

Location: On a line directly below the pupils when looking straight ahead, parallel to the corner of the mouth.

How to find: See illustration of Stomach Meridian (Fig. 2–13).

Technique: Press hard and inward with the index finger for 5–7 seconds, three times.

For: Toothache, facial tension, general tension.

Stomach #6   Kyo Shya (not on chart)

Location: On the hinge of the jaw, on each side of the mouth.

How to find: Have the patient tighten his jaw. You will be able to feel an indentation at the corner of the jaw, slightly in from the jawbone.

Technique: Press softly and inward with one thumb, gradually for 5–7 seconds, three times.

For: Toothache.

Stomach #9   Jin Gei ("welcome human")

Location: One and a half inches from the middle line on the larynx, where a small pulse is felt.

How to find: With the thumb and middle finger of either hand, trace the crease line under your chin until you feel the larynx. Now press in

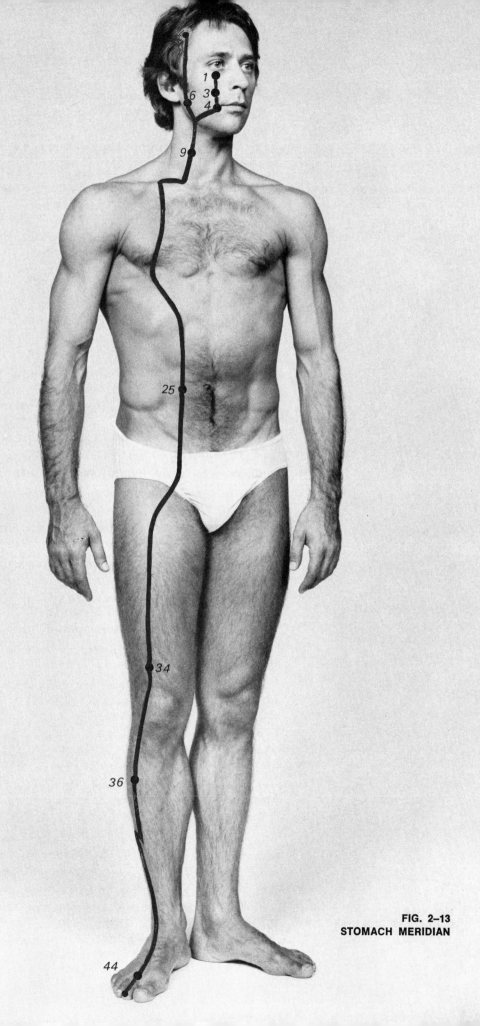

FIG. 2—13
STOMACH MERIDIAN

and slightly away from the larynx. You will feel a pulse on one side of the Adam's apple which marks the correct spot.

Technique: Press softly and inward with one thumb for 10–15 seconds, three times.

For: High blood pressure, beautifying the face.

Stomach #25   Ten Su

Location: Two inches to either lateral side of the navel.

How to find: See illustration of Stomach Meridian (Fig. 2–13).

Technique: Press inward and deeply with three fingers, gradually for 10–15 seconds, three times.

For: Abdominal pain, diarrhea.

Stomach #34   Ryo Kyu ("on the hill")

Location: In the muscle that runs on the outside of the thigh, two inches up from the kneecap.

How to find: Have the patient sit on a chair and bend his leg at a 90-degree angle. Measure two inches up from the top of the kneecap. The point is slightly to the outside of the leg.

Technique: Press hard and inward with one thumb for 7–10 seconds, three times.

For: Stomach pains, diarrhea, arthritis in the knee.

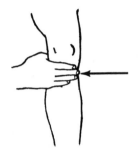

FIG. 2–14
FINDING STOMACH #36

Stomach #36   Ashi San Ri ("three miles")

Location: Bend the patient's leg to 90-degree angle and have him catch his kneecap between index finger and thumb. The middle finger is on the outside of the shinbone, and Stomach #36 is at the tip of this finger (Fig. 2–14).

Technique: Press hard and inward with two thumbs for 10–15 seconds, three times.

For: General well-being, tired legs.

Stomach #44   Nai Tei ("inner garden")

Location: Between second and third toes in the groove of the depression near the second toe bone.

How to find: See illustration of Stomach Meridian (Fig. 2–13).

Technique: Press hard and upward with one thumb for 7–10 seconds, three times.

For: Stomach pain, toothache.

4. SPLEEN MERIDIAN (Yin) Fig. 2–15

Spleen #6   San Yin Ko
("the meeting point of the three Yin leg meridians")

Location: Flex the patient's foot and put his four fingers on the inside of his leg with the little finger resting on top of the anklebone and the other fingers going up the leg. Where the fourth finger lies, behind the shinbone, is Spleen #6 (Fig. 2–16).

Technique: Press hard and inward toward the shinbone with two thumbs for 7–10 seconds, three times.

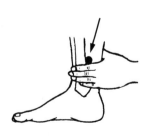

FIG. 2–16
FINDING SPLEEN #6

28

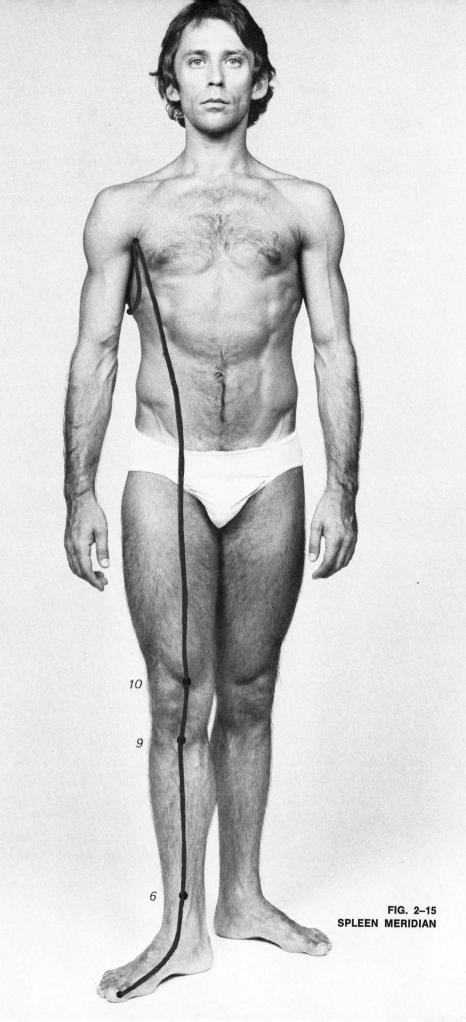

10

9

6

FIG. 2–15
SPLEEN MERIDIAN

For: Pain in the ankles, insomnia, overweight, digestive problems, menstrual pain, any female sexual problem.

When you stimulate Spleen #6 you stimulate the Spleen, Liver, and Kidney meridians.

Spleen #9   Yin Ryo Sen ("Yin mountain pond")

Location: At the top of the shinbone, on the inside of the leg.
How to find: See illustration of Spleen Meridian (Fig. 2–15).
Technique: Press hard and inward with one thumb for 7–10 seconds, three times.
For: Pains in the knee.

Spleen #10   Ketsu Kai ("ocean of blood")

Location: Have the patient sit and bend his leg at a 90-degree angle. Catch the center of his kneecap with the center of your palm. The tip of your thumb will touch Spleen #10, two inches above the kneecap.
Technique: Press hard and inward with one thumb for 5–7 seconds, three times.
For: Itching, neurodermatitis, hives, menstrual pain.

5. HEART MERIDIAN (Yin) Fig. 2–17

In the Orient we believe that fighting spirit resides in the heart. Since the Heart Meridian ends at the little finger, damage to this finger will have an adverse effect on the heart and on the person's fighting spirit. For this reason in olden days when Japanese gangsters were caught, they were forced to cut off their little fingers to guarantee society they would no longer commit violent or aggressive acts.

Heart #3   Shyo Kai ("young ocean") (not on chart)

Location: On the indentation near the inside elbow fold next to the tendon on the inside of the upper arm.
Technique: Press hard and inward with one thumb for 5–7 seconds, three times.
For: Heart palpitations.

Heart #7   Shin Mon ("gate of god")

Location: In the crease on the side of the wrist nearest the little finger.
How to find: Find the bony knob at the base of the outside of the palm. Now have the patient make a tight fist and bend the hand inward. Heart #7 is the small indentation below and slightly to the inside of the wristbone.
Technique: Press hard and inward with one thumb for 5–7 seconds, three times.
For: Reviving an unconscious patient, insomnia, irritability, constipation.

6. SMALL INTESTINE MERIDIAN (Yang) Fig. 2–18

Small Intestine #3   Go Kei ("rear groove")

Location: On the fold that appears when the hand is making a fist, behind the little finger (Fig. 2–19).

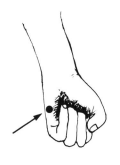

**FIG. 2–19
FINDING SMALL
INTESTINE #3**

30

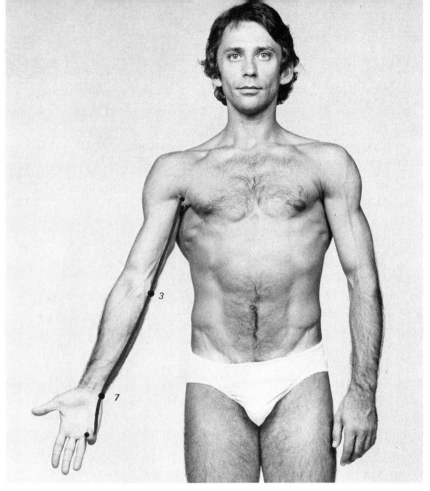

FIG. 2–17
HEART MERIDIAN

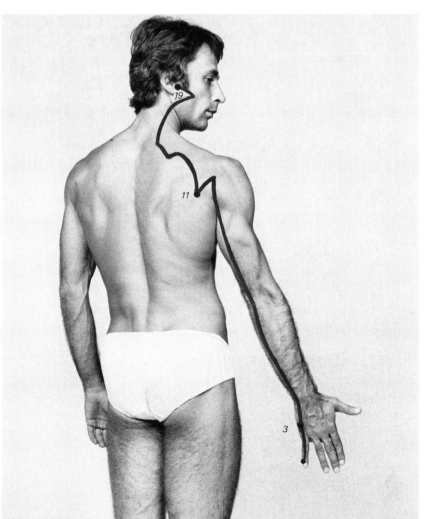

FIG. 2–18
SMALL INTESTINE MERIDIAN

How to find: Open your hand and look at the line that runs across the top of your palm. When you make a fist this line becomes a deep crease. The end of the crease near the little finger is the point for Small Intestine #3.

Technique: Press hard and inward with thumb or pointed object for 7–10 seconds, three times.

For: Numbness and paralysis of fingers.

Small Intestine #11   Ten So

Location: Point is on the horizontal line between the fourth and fifth thoracic vertebrae, in the middle of the "triangle" created by the shoulder blade. (See chapter 4, Back Shiatsu, for vertebrae location.) You can feel a depression where the tsubo is located.

Technique: Press gently and in toward the spine with one thumb for 10–15 seconds, three times. Rotate your thumb, as the point may be very sensitive.

For: Shoulder pain, neuralgia.

Small Intestine #19   Chyo Ku ("palace of hearing")

Location: When you open your mouth an indentation appears just in front of the middle of the ear. If you open and close your mouth you can feel more clearly the indentation where Small Intestine #19 is found.

For: Ringing in the ears.

7. BLADDER MERIDIAN (Yang) Fig. 2–20

There are sixty-seven tsubos in the Bladder Meridian, which begins in the face, runs down the back, and ends in the legs. Bladder Meridian tsubos #11–26 are located between the vertebrae, about one and a half inches to either side of the spine. Bladder #27, #28, and #32 are located on the first, second, and third sacral foramen, or grooves in the sacrum. Many of the bladder points in the back are Associated Points, *Yu*, connected to other organs; the Associated Points are explained in detail, as are pressing techniques, in chapter 4, Back Shiatsu. All of the Bladder Meridian tsubos in the back and hips are pressed the same way, hard and inward with two thumbs for 5–7 seconds, three times. In this chapter I will give only the names of the Bladder Meridian points on the back, their anatomical locations, and the reasons for pressing them. For vertebrae locations see chapter 4.

Bladder #1   Sei Mei ("bright light")

Location: Just outside of tear duct, in the crease at the inner corner of the eye.

Technique: Press hard and inward at 45-degree angle with one thumb or index finger for 10–15 seconds, three times.

For: Poor or tired vision, swollen eyes.

Bladder #10   Ten Chu ("pillar of heaven")

Location: Just below the first cervical vertebra.

How to find: See illustration of Bladder Meridian (Fig. 2–20). One and a half inches lateral to Governing Vessel #15 with Gall Bladder #20 on the other side.

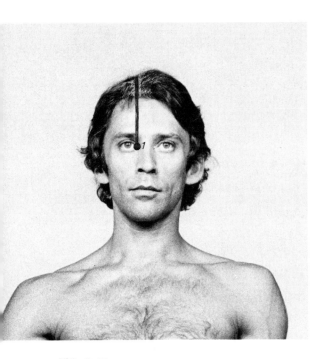

**FIG. 2–20
BLADDER MERIDIAN
(FRONT AND BACK)**

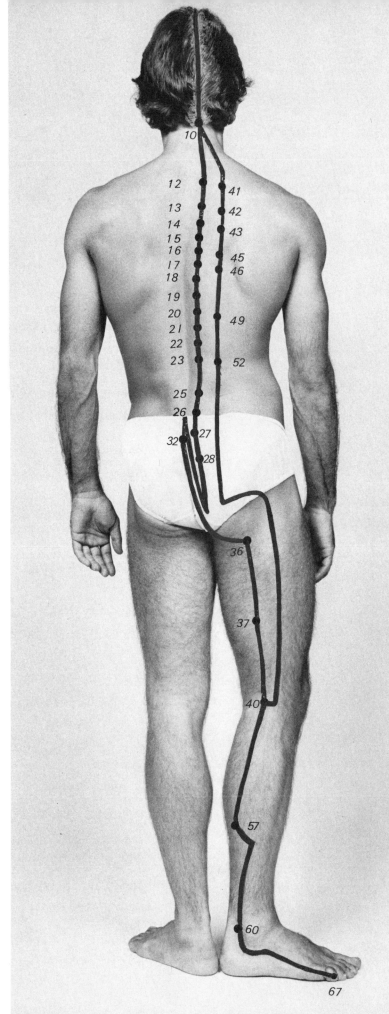

33

Technique: Press with one thumb, avoiding any sudden pressure, for 7–10 seconds, three times.

For: Headache, nasal obstruction.

Bladder #12   Fu Mon ("gate of wind")

Location: One and a half inches on either side of spinal process (or the bones which form the knobby part of the vertebrae) between second and third thoracic vertebrae.

For: Coughing, asthma, any kind of breathing problem.

Bladder #13   Hai Yu (Lung Associated Point)

Location: Between third and fourth thoracic vertebrae.
For: Breathing problems.

Bladder #14   Ketsu Yin Yu
(Heart Constrictor Associated Point)

Location: Between fourth and fifth thoracic vertebrae.
For: Stimulating Conception Vessel Meridian.

Bladder #15   Shin Yu (Heart Associated Point)

Location: Between fifth and sixth thoracic vertebrae, behind the nipple line.
For: Irritability, weak heart.

Bladder #16   Toku Yu (Governing Vessel Associated Point)

Location: Between sixth and seventh thoracic vertebrae.
For: Stimulating Governing Vessel Meridian.

Bladder #18   Kan Yu (Liver Associated Point)

Location: Between ninth and tenth thoracic vertebrae.
For: Liver-associated problems.

Bladder #19   Tan Yu (Gall Bladder Associated Point)

Location: Between tenth and eleventh thoracic vertebrae.
For· Gall-bladder-associated problems.

Bladder #20   Hi Yu (Spleen Associated Point)

Location: Between eleventh and twelfth thoracic vertebrae.
For: Spleen-(pancreas-) associated problems.

Bladder #21   I Yu (Stomach Associated Point)

Location: Between twelfth thoracic and first lumbar vertebrae.
For: Stomach problems.

Bladder #22   San Shyo Yu (Triple Heater Associated Point)

Location: Between first and second lumbar vertebrae.
For: Poor circulation, diarrhea, exhaustion, lower-back ache.

Bladder #23   Jin Yu (Kidney Associated Point)

Location: Between second and third lumbar vertebrae, just behind the navel.

For: Vitalizing patient's energy; kidney-associated problems.

Bladder #25   Dai Cho Yu (Large Intestine Associated Point)

Location: Between fourth and fifth lumbar vertebrae.
For: Large-intestine-associated problems; constipation.

Bladder #26   Kan Gen Yu

Location: Between fifth lumbar vertebra and pelvic bone (see chapter 8 for explanation on how to find).
For: Lower-back ache, digestion, sexual strength.

Bladder #27   Sho Cho Yu (Small Intestine Associated Point)

Location: First groove in sacrum.
For: Small-intestine-related problems.

Bladder #32   Gi Ryo ("second hole")

Location: Second groove in sacrum.
For: Bed-wetting, menstrual irregularities.

Bladder #36   Sho Fu

Location: At base of hip at thighbone.
Technique: Press deeply and inward with one thumb for 7–10 seconds.
For: Sciatica, lower-back ache.

Bladder #37   I Mon

Location: At the midline of the back of thigh, six inches from the fold near the buttocks muscles, halfway between Bladder #36 and Bladder #40.
Technique: Press hard and up with two thumbs for 10–15 seconds, three times.
For: Sciatica, tired legs.

Bladder #40   I Chu

Location: On back of knee, on fold where knee bends, between the two tendons.
Technique: Press softly and inward with two thumbs for 7–10 seconds, three times.
For: Sciatica, lower-back ache, calf spasms.

Bladder Meridian points #41–52 run parallel to points #11–23. They are located between the vertebrae, but three inches on either side of the spinal process, just off the long muscles that run down the back on both sides. Press the same way that you pressed #11–23.

Bladder #41   Fu Bun

Location: Between second and third thoracic vertebrae.
For: Dowager's hump, back curved by age.

Bladder #42   Haku Ko

Location: Between third and fourth thoracic vertebrae.
For: Neck and shoulder pains, cough.

Bladder #43   Ko Ko

Location: Between fourth and fifth thoracic vertebrae.
For: Poor circulation, asthma.

Bladder #45   I Ki

Location: Between sixth and seventh thoracic vertebrae.
For: Fevers, sweating, cough.

Bladder #46   Kaku Kan

Location: Between seventh and eighth thoracic vertebrae.
For: Nausea, vomiting, hiccups.

Bladder #49   I Sha

Location: Between eleventh and twelfth thoracic vertebrae.
For: Diarrhea, stomach ache, tension.

Bladder #52   Shi Shitsu ("chamber of spirits")

Location: Between second and third lumbar vertebrae.
For: Lower-back ache, low energy, kidney trouble.

Bladder #57   Shyo Zan ("in the mountain")

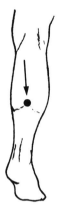

**FIG. 2–21
FINDING BLADDER #57**

Location: Have the patient rise on the balls of his feet. The calf muscle will be easy to see. Bladder #57 is at the beginning of the bulge of the muscle (Fig. 2–21).
Technique: Press softly and inward with one thumb for 10–15 seconds, three times.
For: Sciatica, muscle spasms, tired legs.

Bladder #60   Kon Ron ("mountain")

Location: Draw a line between the outer tip of the base of the ankle-bone and the Achilles tendon. Bladder #60 is at the midpoint.
Technique: Press hard and inward with one thumb for 7–10 seconds, three times.
For: Sciatica, dizziness, epilepsy.

Bladder #67   Shi Yin (extreme Yin) (not on chart)

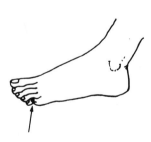

**FIG. 2–22
FINDING BLADDER #67**

Location: On the outside of the little toe, one-tenth of an inch from the lower corner of the nail.
How to find: See Fig. 2–22.
Technique: Press with pointed object, drawing a tiny drop of blood.
For: Easy labor.

8. KIDNEY MERIDIAN (Yin) Fig. 2–23

Kidney #1   Yu Sen ("gushing spring")

Location: On the sole of the foot, slightly less than one-third the distance from the tip of the middle toe to the heel, and midway across the ball of the foot.
How to find: Gently squeeze the top of the patient's foot so that a vertical line appears down the center of the sole. Now fold toes down-

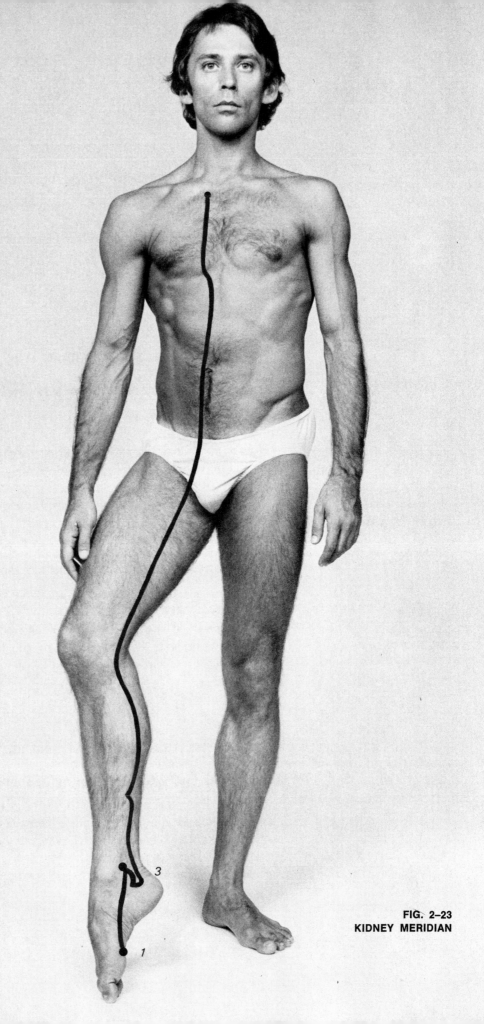

FIG. 2–23
KIDNEY MERIDIAN

ward. A horizontal line will appear. The point at which these two lines intersect is Kidney #1.

Technique: Press hard and inward with two thumbs for 10–15 seconds, three times.

For: Epilepsy, dizziness, menstrual pain, revival.

Kidney #3 Tai Kei ("great groove") (not on chart)

Location: On inside anklebone one-half distance between Achilles tendon and the tip of the anklebone.

How to find: See Kidney Meridian (Fig. 2–23) and feel for the pulse that marks the point.

Technique: Press hard and inward with one thumb for 7–10 seconds, three times.

For: Kidney malfunctions.

9. HEART CONSTRICTOR MERIDIAN (Yin) Fig. 2–24

Heart Constrictor #6 Nai Kan ("inside gate")

Location: Two inches above the wrist fold, in between the two tendons in the wrist.

How to find: Have the patient bend his hand backward. The two tendons will be easy to locate. Now measure about two inches up the arm from the wrist fold.

Technique: Press hard and inward with one thumb for 7–10 seconds, three times.

For: Nausea, vomiting, insomnia, palpitations.

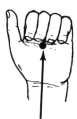

**FIG. 2–25
FINDING HEART
CONSTRICTOR #8**

Heart Constrictor #8 Ro Kyu ("palace of anxiety")

Location: On the palm where the tip of the completely flexed middle finger touches the last crease of the palm.

How to find: The patient bends four fingers to touch the palm. The point is between the tips of the middle and ring fingers (Fig. 2–25).

Technique: Press hard and inward with one thumb for 10–15 seconds, three times.

For: Exhaustion.

10. TRIPLE HEATER MERIDIAN (Yang) Fig. 2–26

Triple Heater #14 Ken Ryo ("top of the shoulder")

Location: Have the patient hold his arm at a 90-degree angle to his body. You will see two indentations on the shoulder, one in front and one in back. Triple Heater #14 is the indentation on the back side. The one in front is Large Intestine #15.

Technique: Press hard and inward with two thumbs for 10–15 seconds, three times.

For: Shoulder joint pains.

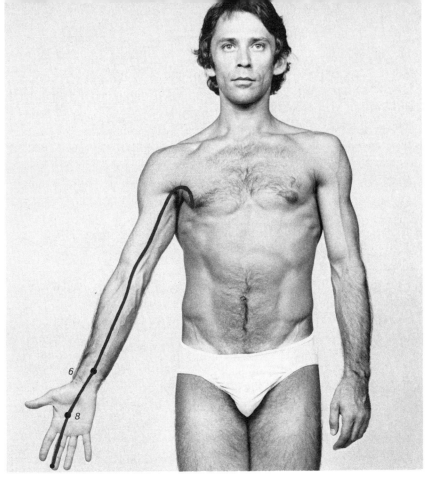

FIG. 2–24
HEART CONSTRICTOR
MERIDIAN

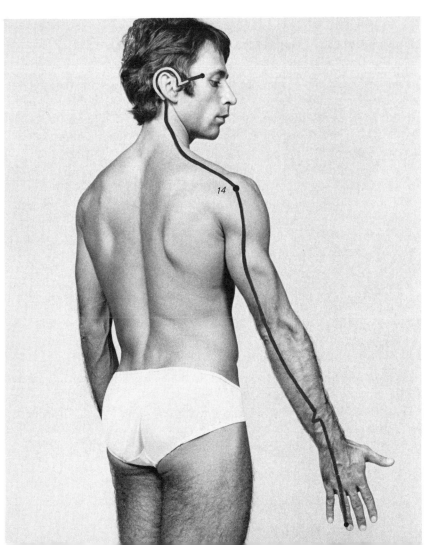

FIG. 2–26
TRIPLE HEATER
MERIDIAN

11. GALL BLADDER MERIDIAN (Yang) Fig. 2–27

Gall Bladder #1   Do Shi Ryo

Location: Next to outer corner of the eye, on the temple.

How to find: See side view illustration on chart and Gall Bladder Meridian (Fig. 2–27).

Technique: Press softly inward with index finger for 10–15 seconds, three times.

For: Eye problems, headache.

Gall Bladder #2   Cho E ("hearing point")

Location: Just below Small Intestine #19.

How to find: When the patient opens his mouth you can feel an indentation on top of the earlobe, slightly in toward the face.

Technique: Press hard and inward with index finger for 7–10 seconds, three times.

For: Ringing in the ears.

Gall Bladder #20   Fu Chi ("pond of wind")

Location: One inch above the hairline, on the sides of the big muscles in the neck.

How to find: See Gall Bladder Meridian (Fig. 2–27).

Technique: Press hard and inward with one thumb for 7–10 seconds, three times.

For: Common cold symptoms, headache, dizziness, swollen eyes.

Gall Bladder #21   Ken Sei ("well in the shoulder")

Location: On shoulder, slightly to the rear.

How to find: Draw a line between the prominent part of the seventh cervical vertebra and the end of the shoulder bone. Gall Bladder #21 is halfway between these points. Or draw a line straight up from the nipple. The point at which it crosses the top of the shoulder is Gall Bladder #21.

Technique: Press firmly but gradually inward with one thumb for 10–15 seconds, three times.

For: Shoulder pain, lack of milk in nursing mothers.

Gall Bladder #24   Jitsu Getsu ("sun and moon")

Location: Between seventh and eighth ribs.

How to find: The point is almost directly below the nipple.

Technique: Press hard and inward with one thumb for 7–10 seconds, three times.

For: Gall bladder ailments.

Gall Bladder #25   Kei Mon ("gate of the capitol")

Location: Just below the twelfth rib on the back, toward the side of the torso.

Technique: Press hard and inward with one thumb for 5–7 seconds, three times.

For: Stomach ache, digestive problems, vomiting.

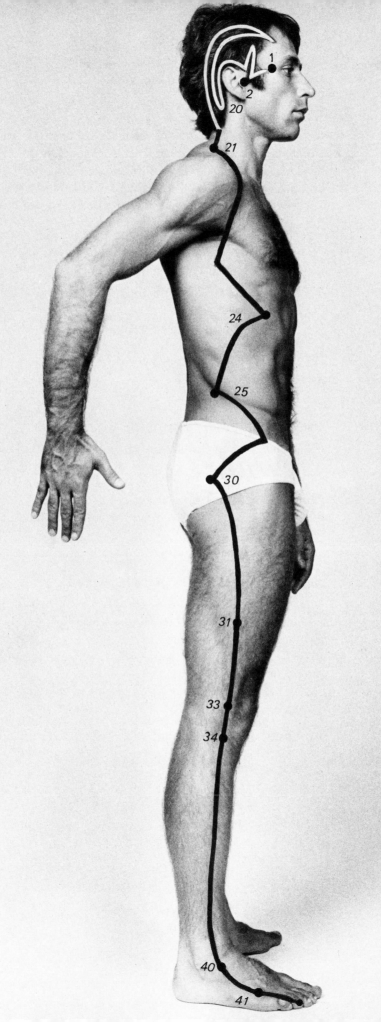

**FIG. 2–27
GALL BLADDER
MERIDIAN**

Gall Bladder #30   Kan Chyo

Location: On the large indentation on the hip.

How to find: You can see the indentation on the side of the hip when the patient stands up straight. You can also find the point by having the patient lie on his side and bend his legs at a 90-degree angle. Make a fist by placing the knuckle of your little finger on the top of the hip. Roll your fist downward; the thumb will fall on Gall Bladder #30.

Technique: Press hard and inward with two thumbs for 10–15 seconds, three times.

For: Sciatica, lower-back ache.

Gall Bladder #31   Fu Shi ("market of wind")

Location: On the side of the thigh at the tip of the middle finger when the arms are straight down.

How to find: The patient stands up and puts his arms at his sides. The point is below the tip of his middle finger.

Technique: Press gradually inward (deeply) with two thumbs for 10–15 seconds, three times.

For: Circulation in legs, tired legs.

Gall Bladder #34   Yo Ryo Sen

Location: Just under the kneecap on the side of the leg.

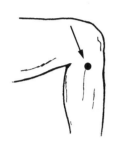

**FIG. 2–28
FINDING GALL
BLADDER #34**

How to find: Have the patient sit on a chair with his legs bent at a 90-degree angle. Gall Bladder #34 is in the bony indentation below and to the outside of the base of the kneecap (Fig. 2–28).

Technique: Press hard and inward with one thumb for 7–10 seconds, three times.

For: Ankle pains, headache.

Gall Bladder #41   Rin Kyu ("almost crying")

Location: In the depression between the fourth and fifth toes.

How to find: Measure two fingers' width up from the bridge between the fourth and fifth toes.

Technique: Press softly and upward with one thumb for 5–10 seconds, three times.

For: Menstrual pain, foot pains, ringing in the ears.

12. LIVER MERIDIAN (Yin) Fig. 2–29

Liver #3   Tai Chu

Location: Measure one and a half inches up from the bridge between the big toe and the second toe.

Technique: Press hard and upward with one thumb for 7–10 seconds, three times.

For: Headaches, dizziness.

Liver #4   Chu Ho

Location: Halfway between the front edge of the anklebone and the stringy muscles at the top of the foot.

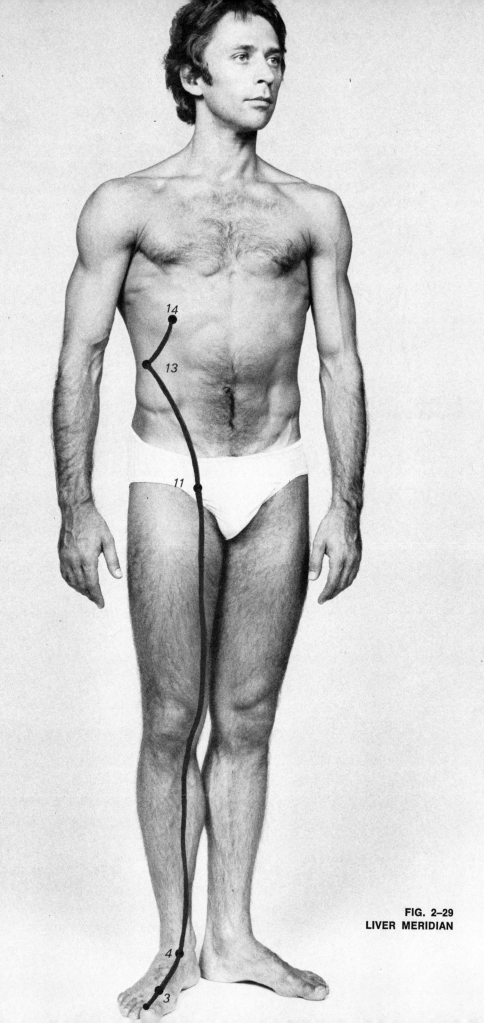

FIG. 2–29
LIVER MERIDIAN

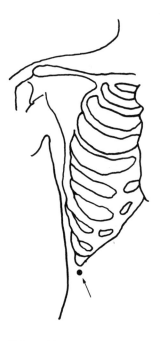

FIG. 2–30
FINDING LIVER #13

Technique: Press hard and inward with one thumb for 7–10 seconds, three times.

For: Arthritis in the ankle, lower-back ache.

Liver #11   In Ren

Location: Two inches down from the crease between the thigh and the torso.

How to find: See Liver Meridian (Fig. 2–29).

Technique: Press hard and inward with one thumb for 7–10 seconds, three times.

For: Menstrual pain, frigidity.

Liver #13   Shyo Mon

Location: Just below the front tip of the rib cage (Fig. 2–30).

Technique: Press hard and inward with one thumb for 7–10 seconds, three times.

For: Abdominal pain, vomiting.

Liver #14   Ki Mon

Location: Between sixth and seventh ribs, directly under the nipple.

How to find: See Liver Meridian (Fig. 2–29).

Technique: Press softly and inward with one thumb for 5–10 seconds, three times.

For: Rib pains, poor lactation in nursing mothers.

13. GOVERNING VESSEL MERIDIAN (Yang) Fig. 2–31

The Governing Vessel Meridian runs between the two rows of Bladder Meridian tsubos and the points are located on the spine between the vertebrae. All of the points on the spine are pressed the same way, in and hard with one thumb, three times.

Governing Vessel #4   Mei Mon ("gate of life")

Location: Between the second and third lumbar vertebrae just behind the navel.

How to find: Wrap a string around the body passing it over the navel. The place where the string crosses the spine is Governing Vessel #4.

For: Lumbar pain, headaches, ringing in the ears, impotence.

Governing Vessel #11   Shin Do ("path of god")

Location: Between fifth and sixth thoracic vertebrae.

For: Stroke.

Governing Vessel #12   Shin Chu ("pillar of body")

Location: Between third and fourth thoracic vertebrae.

For: Asthma, colds.

Governing Vessel #14   Dai Tsui ("big vertebra")

Location: Between seventh cervical vertebra and first thoracic vertebra.

For: Fever, headaches, cold, allergies, asthma.

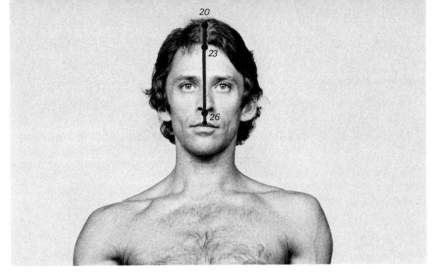

FIG. 2–31
GOVERNING VESSEL
MERIDIAN
(FRONT AND BACK)

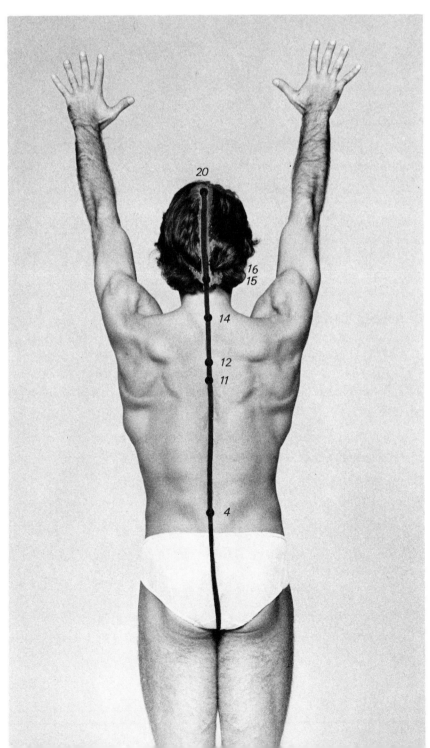

Governing Vessel #15   A Mon ("gate of fool")

Location: On the midline of the neck, one-half inch above the hairline, between first and second cervical vertebrae.

Technique: Press inward and upward with one thumb for 7–10 seconds, three times.

For: Headaches, nosebleeds, colds.

Governing Vessel #16   Fu Fu ("capitol of wind")

Location: One inch above the hairline at the center of the neck.

How to find: One-half inch above Governing Vessel #15.

Technique: Press hard, inward and upward, with one thumb for 7–10 seconds, three times.

For: Common colds, strokes.

Governing Vessel #20   Hya Kue ("one hundred meetings")

Location: In the middle of the line connecting the upper edge of the two ears, at the center of the head (Fig. 2–32).

Technique: Press hard and downward with two thumbs for 10–15 seconds, three times.

For: Headaches, heatstroke, hemorrhoids.

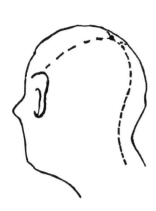

**FIG. 2–32
FINDING GOVERNING
VESSEL #20**

Governing Vessel #23   Jo Sei ("upper star")

Location: One inch behind the front hairline (or original hairline, if there is balding).

How to find: Put the wrist line of the patient's hand on the end of his nose. The tip of his middle finger will touch the tsubo.

Technique: Press hard and inward with the two thumbs for 7–10 seconds, three times.

For: Headaches and nasal problems.

Governing Vessel #26   Nin Chu ("center of human")

Location: One-third the distance down from the end of the nostrils to the edge of the upper lip.

How to find: See Governing Vessel Meridian (Fig. 2–31).

Technique: Press hard and inward with index finger or a pointed object for 7–10 seconds, three times.

For: Loss of consciousness, epilepsy.

14. CONCEPTION VESSEL MERIDIAN (Yin) Fig. 2–33

Conception Vessel #4   Kan Gen ("gate of origin")

Location: In the middle of the abdomen, three inches below the navel.

How to find: See Conception Vessel Meridian (Fig. 2–33) and chapter 5, Ampuku Therapy.

Technique: Press inward, gradually and deeply, with palm of hand for 10–15 seconds, three times.

For: Menstrual cramps, frigidity, impotency.

Conception Vessel #6   Ki Kai ("ocean of ki-energy")

Location: In the middle of the abdomen, one and a half inches below the navel.

FIG. 2–33
CONCEPTION VESSEL
MERIDIAN

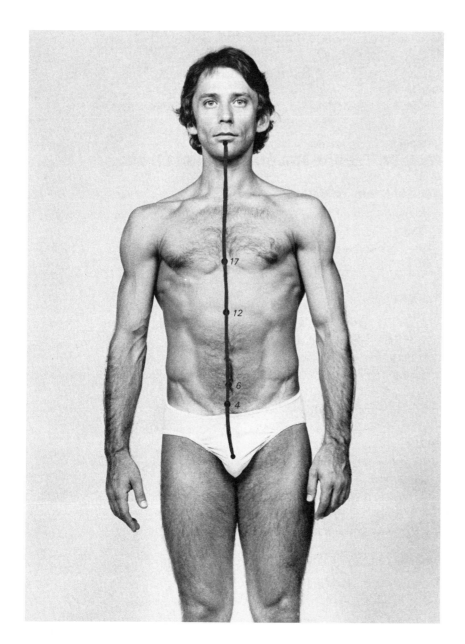

Technique: Press inward, gradually and deeply, with palm of hand for 10–15 seconds, three times.

For: Stomach pain, diarrhea, wet dreams, menstrual pain, constipation.

Conception Vessel #12 Chu Kan ("midway")

Location: In the middle of the abdomen, four inches above the navel, midway between the navel and the pit of the stomach, or solar plexus.

Technique: Press downward and inward, softly, with palm of hand for 10–15 seconds, three times.

For: Nausea, vomiting, diarrhea.

Conception Vessel #17 Dan Chu

Location: Middle of the sternum, at the level of the nipples.

How to find: Draw a line from one nipple to the other nipple. The point

47

is at the place where this line intersects with the line that runs down the middle of the sternum.

Technique: Press softly inward with two thumbs for 10–15 seconds, three times.

For: Asthma, high blood pressure, lack of milk in nursing women.

Special Tsubos Not on Meridian Lines

Ten Shi ("joint point")

Location: About three inches from the hipbone, in toward the buttocks.
How to find: See chart.
Technique: Press inward toward the spine.
For: Sciatica, numbness in the legs, lower-back ache, sexual strength.

Tai Yo ("sun")

Location: One finger's width to the side of the eyebrow, between the end of the eyebrow and the outer edge of the eye.
How to find: See chart.
Technique: Press inward with one thumb gradually and hard for 7–10 seconds, three times.
For: Headaches, red, swollen eyes, dizziness.

In Do

Location: Between the eyebrows on the Governing Vessel Meridian.
How to find: See chart.
Technique: Press hard and inward with two thumbs for 7–10 seconds, three times.
For: Headaches, nasal obstruction.

Ohashi's point

See chapter 6, Neck Shiatsu.

3. Shiatsu Technique

A few days after I finished my Shiatsu training in Tokyo I was called in by an older gentleman who wanted a treatment. Without a word I began working on him. A few moments passed and then he said, "I don't need you. Go home!"

"Why?" I asked, quite startled. His reply was, "You are still a novice, just starting your career, and not yet a therapist. I asked for a Shiatsu therapist."

I told him that he was correct and that I had only begun my career a few days before. How did he know? How could he tell? I hadn't told him a thing about myself.

He said, "Listen, young man. I've been taking Shiatsu treatments for more than thirty years, long before you were born. I can tell by the first touch whether or not someone knows Shiatsu. I can tell if they have talent or not, what school they attended, their experience, and everything else I need to know. You may have been silent, but your fingers were not."

The Shiatsu practitioner, of course, owes most of his skill to experience. It is also true that Shiatsu is not merely a manipulative technique; the practitioner's attitude plays a large role in the quality of the treatment. If you have no empathy with your patient, your Shiatsu is worthless.

In Shiatsu we use no machines, no oils, no equipment; we use only our hands. Hands are a part of our own human body and easily reflect our emotions. If you are nervous, for example, your hands become tense and sweaty. They cannot move smoothly if you have bad feelings for your patient. I therefore prefer to work only on people I like, and judging from my experience, these positive feelings produce the best Shiatsu. After giving Shiatsu to someone I like I feel less tired and the patient is happy and satisfied.

It is wonderful to practice Shiatsu in your family circle because Shiatsu is such an excellent form of communication. If all families were to practice Shiatsu, there would be less family conflict, smaller generation gaps, and more happiness, health, love, and peace on earth.

When and Where to Give Shiatsu

Since we use no equipment in Shiatsu we can work anywhere, anytime —the desert, the beach, a mountaintop—wherever we may be. One of the best places to give Shiatsu, however, is on a carpeted floor. The firmness of the floor makes it easier for the practitioner to bring the weight of his body into the tsubo he is pressing. When you are working on the patient's back, have him lie flat on his stomach with his face turned sideways. Never place a pillow under his head, as this may produce muscle spasms when you apply pressure to the neck and shoulders. The patient's arms should be at his sides and he should not cradle his head in his arms, as this position prevents him from relaxing fully. His rib cage must rest flat and even on the floor, or else he will feel uncomfortable and you will risk injuring the rib cage. When you are working on the patient's stomach he must lie on his back with his arms at his sides and a pillow under his head. In both positions the patient's mouth should be slightly open and the eyes closed for greater relaxation.

The treatment room must be clean, quiet, and warm. The subject must be comfortable and relaxed because when the body is rigid, a barrier is created which prevents any healing from taking place.

Breathing

Relaxation is achieved by a proper breathing pattern. In Shiatsu it is important to apply pressure only when the patient is exhaling. When he is inhaling, his body becomes harder and tighter and to give pressure at this time would produce much discomfort and could cause muscle spasms, as well as eliminating all possible benefits of the treatment. Watch for the rise and fall of the chest or back (depending on how he is lying), or if you are inexperienced say, "Breathe in, breathe out." Orthopedists and chiropractors use the same method.

Precautions

1. Know the body of the person you are working on. Diagnosis of a patient, from either an Oriental or Western viewpoint, is a highly complicated procedure, and as an amateur Shiatsu therapist you should not rely solely on your own judgment. If you know or suspect a patient is seriously ill, don't give Shiatsu without having him or her consult a physician. Remember, the main purpose of Shiatsu, especially that given by the amateur practitioner, is not to cure disease but to help someone recover from the fatigue and strain of daily routines, or to relieve symptoms of disease, or to prevent it.

2. Don't give Shiatsu when your patient is very hungry or very full after eating a big meal. Wait at least two hours. If you have a very hungry patient, wait until he has had a little to eat.

3. If your patient is very tired, sweating heavily, or has a fast heartbeat, wait until all is normal.

4. Don't treat patients with broken or fractured bones.

5. Don't treat patients with contagious diseases (such as osteomyelitis, measles, whooping cough, or flu with fever); with any disorders of the heart, liver, kidneys, or lungs; or with cancer, sarcoma, or infectious skin

diseases. Remember, serious illness can be cured by Shiatsu, but only by an experienced Shiatsu therapist with an excellent knowledge of diagnostic procedure and other forms of Oriental medicine.

When to Have Shiatsu

If you are planning to take Shiatsu, the time and place is when and where you most enjoy it. Preferably, you should receive Shiatsu in a situation where the temperature is moderate and the atmosphere quiet and relaxing. In general, you can take Shiatsu once a day at any time. If you've just had a bath, you should rest a half hour before beginning the treatment. A session should last about thirty minutes, but overtreatment is better than no treatment at all. Quality (pressing the right tsubos correctly using a proper technique) is always better than quantity. Be sure to rest a while after the treatment.

While taking Shiatsu you should relax and give in completely to the practitioner's pressure. This is possible only if you are inhaling and exhaling in a relaxed and regular pattern.

Yin and Yang Shiatsu

According to Shiatsu diagnosis, patients can be placed into two categories—Yin and Yang. The Yin patient we call "empty," underfunctioning. In order to "tonify," or increase the energy level of the Yin patient, the practitioner must give him energy or tonify the patient's own energy within his body; and for this he must be Yang, healthier than the patient. In tonification technique you must (1) work in the direction of the energy flow in the meridian, or begin with the first tsubo in the meridian and press all tsubos consecutively till you reach the last tsubo; and (2) work slowly and gently.

The Yang patient is too "full," overfunctioning. In treating him, you have to draw out his excess energy through a sedation technique. In sedation technique you (1) work against the meridian, or begin pressing the last tsubo and work your way to the first, in the opposite direction of the energy flow; and (2) apply quick, strong pressure.

It is not easy to tell if a patient is Yin or Yang. Generally, you can tell by looking at him and observing his behavior. Fat people with well-developed muscle structures are often Yang; and slender, or flabby people, Yin. Vigorous, active people are Yang, and weak, listless people are Yin. The same person can be Yin or Yang at different times. One day you may feel weak and tired (Yin) and the next day strong and active (Yang). Occasionally, however, a person may seem to be Yin or Yang externally and yet be the opposite on the inside. One of the best and surest ways to diagnose a patient as Yin or Yang is to take his pulse Oriental-style (an advanced technical procedure, much too complicated to explain here) and determine the flow of energy through the meridian lines. Usually, though, appearances are reliable and your intuition will suffice.

In general, people who are dealing with health must be healthy. Sick people hesitate to be treated by a sick doctor. Especially when you are giving Yin Shiatsu you must transfer your energy to the patient. If you are not healthy and don't have enough energy, your patient could weaken you and you could become more tired, or drained of energy.

Character of the Fingers

The fingers (including the thumbs) are our main tools in Shiatsu, and their sensitivity and effectiveness are extremely important. Some Shiatsu specialists in Japan go so far as to take insurance on their thumbs and fingers, for obvious reasons. Some people have good fingers to begin with, others don't, but to a large extent, everyone's fingers strengthen and develop through doing Shiatsu. It is important to keep your fingers in good shape both by using them correctly and by doing exercises to develop them, which I describe later in this chapter.

In Japan we divide the Shiatsu practitioner's fingers into two categories: (1) *karate*, literally meaning "bitter"—karate fingers are hard but strong, they are painful but effective, especially for the sedation technique required by Yang-type patients, and (2) *amate*, literally meaning "sweet." Amate fingers are soft, but comfortable, good for giving the Yin-type patient tonification. I have amate fingers—comfortable but penetrating. Generally speaking, it is better to have amate-type hands than karate-type.

The ideal Shiatsu therapist has big hands and a small body. The bigger the hands and the smaller the body, the better for giving Shiatsu, as one of my teachers used to say. After you've been practicing for a long time, your hands will enlarge and become softer. When you do Shiatsu your hands should be warm, because the patient will find a chilly hand very uncomfortable. Be sure to cut your nails short to avoid scratching the patient, but leave the corner of the nail intact to keep it strong.

Correct Use and Development of the Thumbs and Fingers

Your thumbs are the most important fingers for Shiatsu. But don't make the mistake of being "all thumbs," and ceasing to use other Shiatsu techniques (such as elbows, fingers, and hands). If you use only your thumbs, they will become swollen and painful. You will tire easily because you are using only one part of your body. As you become uncomfortable, you will communicate your discomfort to the patient, who will perceive it and become uneasy. The treatment will be less effective.

Usually you need to press each tsubo with only one thumb, but at certain times you might need more pressure, which you can achieve by pressing while holding one thumb on top of the other. Use the ball or flat of the thumb, never the tip, to press. Apply pressure steadily without jiggling or rubbing. Pressing with the tips or rubbing while pressing can injure the thumbs and fingers and damage the person you are treating. Again, trim all long nails, making sure they don't extend over the top of the thumb (Figs. 3–1, 3–2, and 3–3).

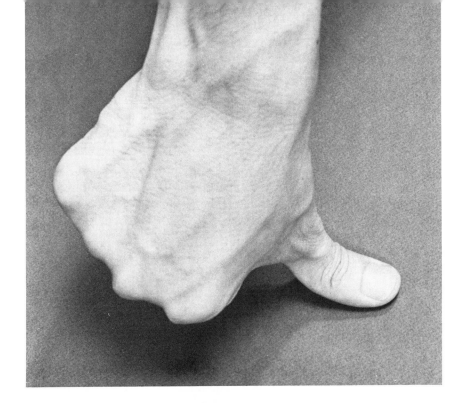

FIG. 3–1
PRESSING WITH
THE THUMB

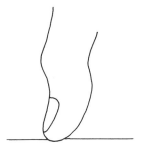

FIG. 3–2
INCORRECT

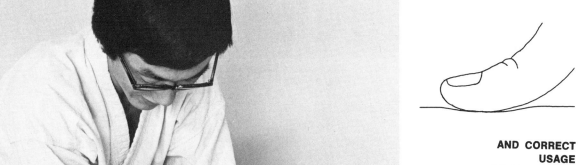

AND CORRECT
USAGE
OF THE THUMB

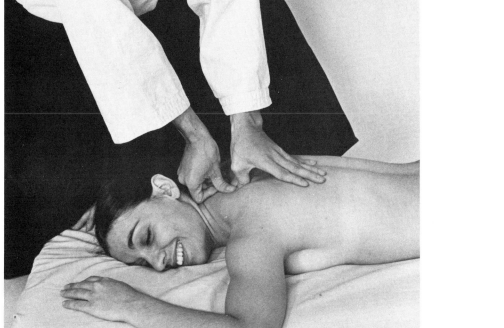

FIG. 3–3
PRESSING WITH
ONE THUMB
ON TOP
OF THE OTHER

HOW TO DEVELOP THE THUMBS

One of the most practical exercises to develop the thumbs and improve the muscle tone in your arms and chest is to press one thumb hard against the other. Do this for a few seconds at first, then gradually increase the amount of time and pressure (Fig. 3–4).

If you want to astonish your friends while developing the strength and penetration ability of your thumbs and arms, do twenty push-ups a day, using just your thumbs to support the weight of your body. I do this exercise every day (Fig. 3–5). Fortunately, it's not the only way to develop the thumbs.

FIG. 3–4
PRESSING ONE THUMB
AGAINST THE OTHER
TO STRENGTHEN THEM

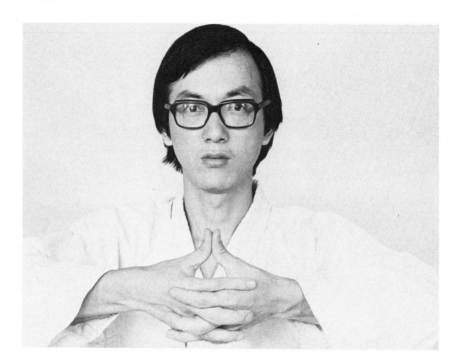

FIG. 3–5
OHASHI DOING PUSH-UPS
USING ONLY HIS THUMBS
TO SUPPORT HIS
BODY WEIGHT

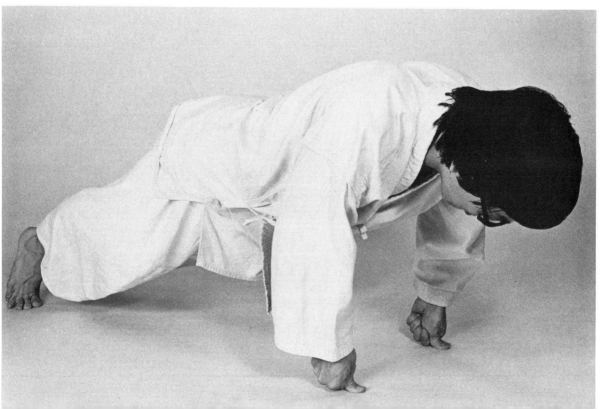

EXERCISES FOR STRENGTHENING THE FINGERS

1. Press one hand against the other with palms flat and all the fingers together (Fig. 3–6).

2. Press one hand against the other, with the thumbs separated from the other fingers (Fig. 3–7).

3. Bend fingers back on each hand, using the other hand (Fig. 3–8).

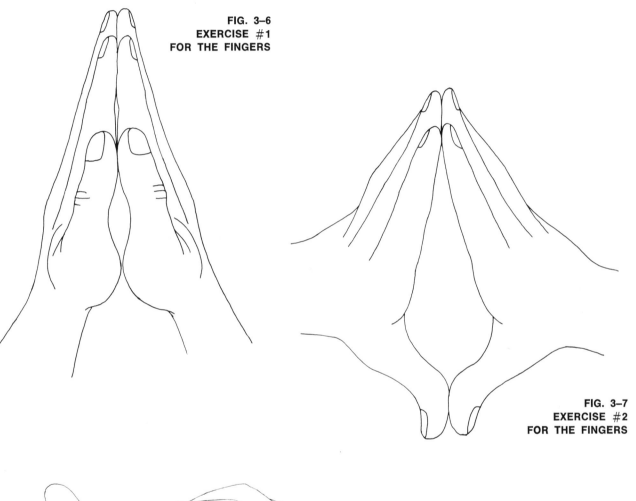

FIG. 3–6
EXERCISE #1
FOR THE FINGERS

FIG. 3–7
EXERCISE #2
FOR THE FINGERS

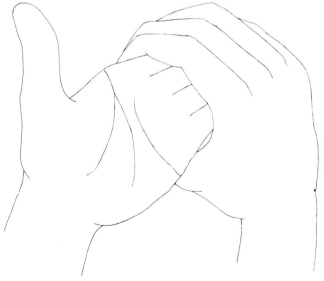

FIG. 3–8
EXERCISE #3
FOR THE FINGERS

Pressing the Tsubo

Never use only your fingertips to press the tsubo. Apply your whole body. You can apply pressure steadily or use a back-and-forth motion, which will give the patient a pleasant, rhythmic Shiatsu. Although I weigh only 112 pounds, I must often work on people who weigh 200 to 250 pounds, especially in America. In such cases I must be able to concentrate my entire body weight on one tsubo in order to give adequate pressure.

When you are pressing, never bend your arms or position your body too far from the patient. If you bring your body close to the patient and keep your elbows straight, you will be able to use the energy from your *Hara*, or central navel area, and make the most efficient use of your weight. If you want to exert what we call "triangle gravity pressure," keep your body erect, then stretch your arms and lean forward. Your weight will be concentrated on the thumbs. Lean on your thumbs and let gravity do the work (Figs. 3–9, 3–10). Again, press only when the patient is exhaling.

THE DIRECTION TO PRESS

The direction in which pressure is applied to each tsubo varies. Generally, you press toward the center of the body. In order to do this you

**FIG. 3–9
KEEP THE ELBOWS STRAIGHT AND BRING THE BODY CLOSE TO THE PATIENT'S; THE PATIENT IS LYING IN THE POSITION CORRECT FOR RECEIVING BACK SHIATSU**

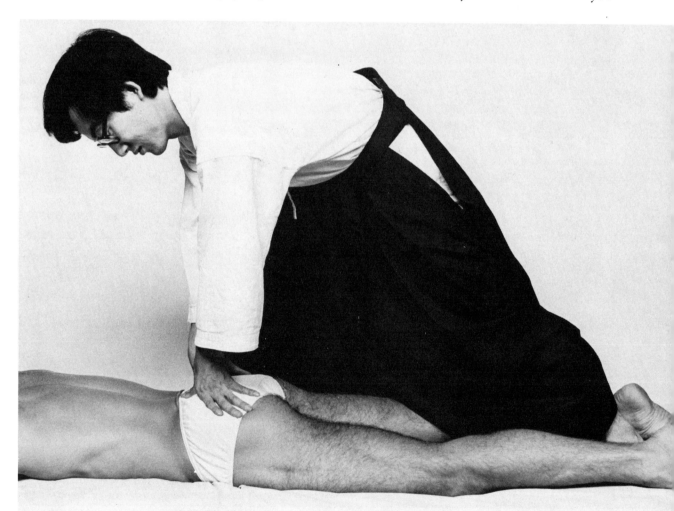

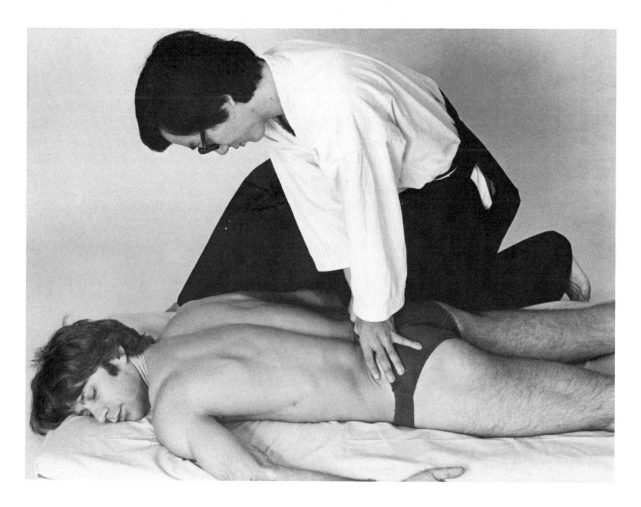

FIG. 3–10
TRIANGLE GRAVITY
PRESSURE

have to evaluate, and often readjust the position of your own body each time you apply pressure. As you know from chapter 2 different tsubos are pressed in different ways. I have made an indication for pressure direction for each tsubo throughout the book. The chart reproduced in chapter 2 is also a useful guide.

HOW LONG TO PRESS

Pressure is generally applied to the tsubo for three to five seconds. When pressing the back tsubo, however, you should press five to seven seconds (count to ten yourself). There are many exceptions to these general guidelines which I note in chapter 2. If the patient complains of sudden, severe pain you should stop pressing at once. Pain can be a signal of serious internal problems, so don't ignore it. Proper pressing on the tsubos gives the patient a sensation somewhere between pleasure and pain. We call this "comfortable pain"; it is the kind of pain the patient can bear easily when he knows the Shiatsu is helping him. If you have any doubts about the quality of the pain or if it seems extremely severe, have the patient consult a doctor for a checkup before proceeding. If this statement sounds vague, it will become less so after you've practiced Shiatsu for a time. No matter how many books you read, charts you consult, or classes you take, there is no substitute for personal experience in the practice of Shiatsu.

Pressing Techniques

PRESSING SLOWLY—RELEASING SLOWLY

This is the most fundamental Shiatsu technique. You should press gradually, adding to the pressure as you watch the patient's face for reactions. Maintain the pressure at its peak for three to five seconds, then release gradually. This is a good technique for relieving muscle spasms and nervous tension and for revitalizing a tired body. It is also a tonification technique for a Yin-type patient.

PRESSING SUDDENLY—RELEASING SUDDENLY

This is a more difficult technique, used by professional therapists who fully understand Shiatsu. You press slowly, then suddenly harder, and release suddenly. It is an effective method to use on the spinal cord and a good sedation technique for Yang-type patients.

PRESSING WITH THE PALM

The palm of the hand is used to apply pressure to the softer spots of the body, such as the eyes and abdomen. Press with the palm or four fingers on the stomach, abdomen, or eyes for about one minute. You can also put one palm on top of the other hand for added pressure. Remember, pressure always comes from your body through your stretched elbow to your relaxed palm. This method relieves pain, burning sensations in the stomach, and tired eyes. It is also tonification for the Yin-type patient.

INDEX FINGER TECHNIQUE

To use the index finger for pressing tsubo, put your middle finger on top of the index finger for a very efficient form of pressure (Figs. 3–11 and 3–12).

FIG. 3–11 (BELOW LEFT) PLACING THE MIDDLE FINGER ON TOP OF THE INDEX FINGER FOR ADDED PRESSURE

FIG. 3–12 (BELOW RIGHT) PLACING THE MIDDLE FINGER ON TOP OF THE INDEX FINGER FOR ADDED PRESSURE

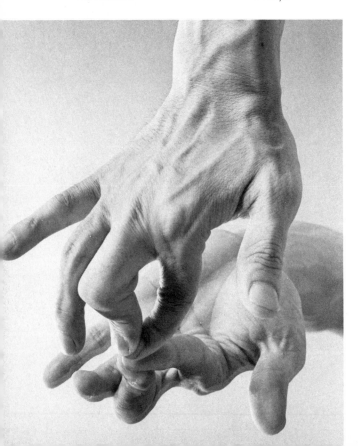
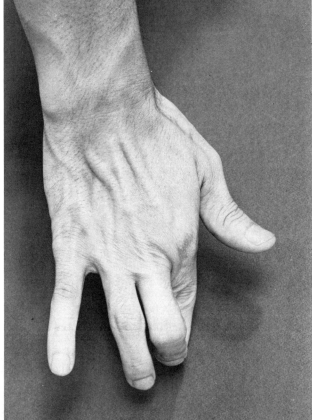

TWO-FINGER TECHNIQUE

If you are applying pressure to wider tsubos (which are located in the back, stomach, hips, and thighs), two fingers—the index and middle finger—used side by side can give a moderate pressure (Fig. 3–13).

Special Shiatsu Techniques

Here are several different techniques to use in a Shiatsu treatment, according to the needs of the individual patient you are working on. In chapter 11 we suggest a complete Shiatsu routine, which includes these techniques and others from later chapters which can be used in a general regimen of Shiatsu to promote and to maintain health and a feeling of well-being.

KENBIKI TECHNIQUE

Kenbiki, one of the most commonly used Shiatsu techniques, loosens and relaxes the muscles and tendons on any part of the patient's body. Kenbiki means "pushing and pulling the muscles," and can be done with the thumbs or fingers. In Fig. 3–14 I am pushing and pulling the muscles along the patient's spine with my thumbs, and in Fig. 3–15 I am using four fingers, with one hand placed on top of the other to give extra pressure. Use Kenbiki before pressing the tsubos.

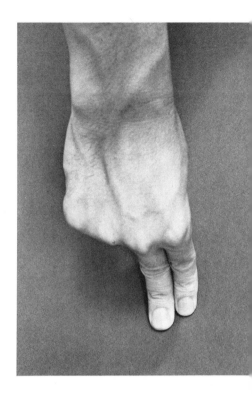

**FIG. 3–13 (ABOVE)
USING TWO FINGERS TO
GIVE MODERATE PRESSURE
ON WIDER TSUBOS**

FIGS. 3–14 AND 3–15   KENBIKI TECHNIQUE

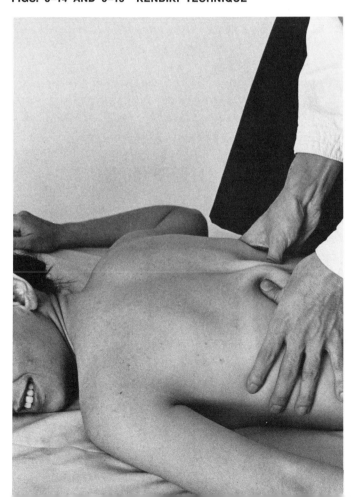

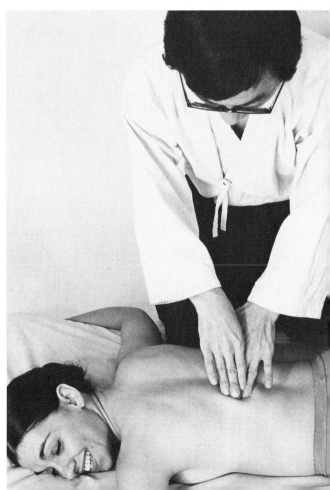

PERCUSSION TECHNIQUES

There are several different percussion movements. For all of them it is important that the practitioner be completely relaxed, making sure there is no tension in his elbows, which will insure relaxed hands and a pleasant treatment for the patient. You should never hit so hard that the patient feels a reverberation in the head. Two or three minutes of percussion is sufficient.

Cupping the hands. Relax the hands completely. Now cup them and tap them all over the patient's back. The tapping should have a quick, light, staccato quality. This may produce a loud noise, but the patient won't find it painful. Do it for two or three minutes on the upper back, lower back, and hips. This is good for improving circulation and relaxing muscles (Fig. 3–16).

Fist percussion technique. Make a loose fist. Hit gently across the shoulders and upper back, lower back (very gently), and the head (slowly, gently) for two to three minutes. Be careful not to hit hard, especially if the patient has high blood pressure (Fig. 3–17).

Double-cushion percussion. Keeping the fingers together and clasping the hands, hit the patient with the back side of one hand. If your hands are loose enough, you will hear the air escaping from between the palms. This technique is good for tired shoulders, muscle tension, poor circulation, and as a general relaxant. Apply softly and slowly for two to three minutes to the head, upper back, lower back, and shoulders (Fig. 3–18).

Percussion with backs of fingers. This technique involves hitting the patient very quickly with the backs of the fingers. Relax the fingers completely. Now, using them like little whips, hit with the backs of the fingers around the head, shoulders, neck, and upper and lower back. Continue down the hips and legs, spending two or three minutes on the entire area (Fig. 3–19).

Here are some additional techniques that are very basic in the practice of Shiatsu. You should first master each one separately and in time work them into a complete Shiatsu. Like the percussion techniques, they help improve circulation and relax tense muscles. Experience will tell you how long to press, how much, and in what direction. Again, let the patient's reaction be your guide. If he feels a "comfortable" pressure, you are applying the technique correctly.

INSERTING THE FINGERS BENEATH THE SHOULDER BLADE

Insert your thumb or three or four fingers beneath the shoulder blade. If the patient is not relaxed, you will not be able to do this. Loosen the shoulder by shaking gently to make the technique easier to perform. You may be able to insert your fingers to their second joints. This is good for frozen shoulder, nervous tension, heart disease, and arm pain (Fig. 3–21).

PUSHING AND PULLING MUSCLES ALONG THE SPINE

Place all of the fingers of one of your hands on one side of the spine and push toward the head. Place the other hand at the same level on the other

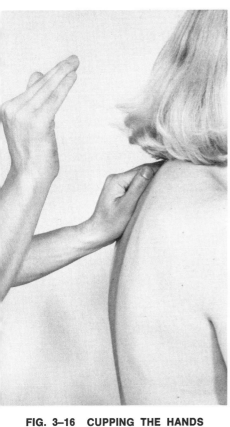

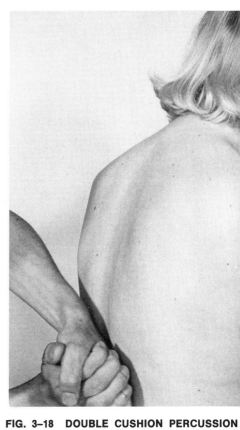

FIG. 3–16 CUPPING THE HANDS   FIG. 3–17 FIST PERCUSSION TECHNIQUE   FIG. 3–18 DOUBLE CUSHION PERCUSSION

FIGS. 3–19
PERCUSSION WITH BACKS OF FINGERS

FIG. 3–20
GRABBING AND LIFTING MUSCLE

FIG. 3–21 INSERTING FINGERS
BENEATH THE SHOULDER BLADE

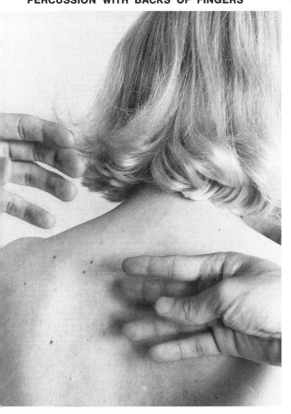

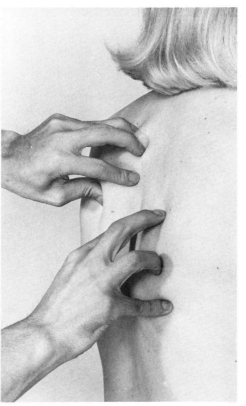

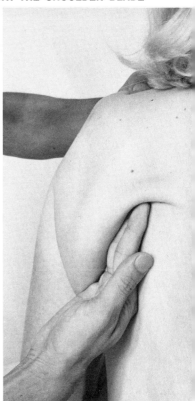

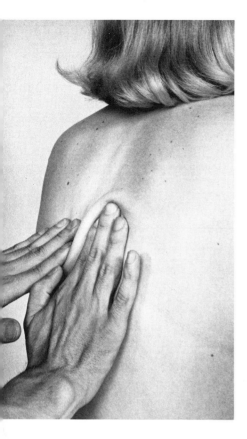

**FIG. 3–22
PUSHING AND PULLING
THE SPINE**

side of the spine and push down. Now push and pull with both hands at the same time and apply the technique all along the spine. This is used to treat muscle spasms and release tension (Fig. 3–22).

USING THE ELBOW ON THE BACK AND THIGHS

The elbow is used to work on muscular areas like the lower back, the hips, and the thighs. The elbow can give stronger pressure, which covers a larger area than the thumbs. Place the elbow over the tsubo and press toward you (Fig. 3–23). A "sharp" elbow (Fig. 3–24) gives a more specific, intense pressure. A more relaxed elbow (Fig. 3–25) gives a more general, milder pressure.

USING THE FIST ALONG THE SPINE

Make a fist and move the hand up and down the sides of the spine along the first Bladder Meridian (Figs. 3–26 and 3–27). This is good for lower-back ache and loosening the back muscles.

PULLING THE BACK MUSCLES

Grab the muscle along the patient's spine between bent index and middle fingers. Pull up. Repeat along the muscular areas of the back, shoulders, neck, and arms to loosen muscles and increase circulation (Fig. 3–28).

KNIFE TECHNIQUE

Take the blade of the hand (as if you were giving a "karate chop") and place the little finger on the muscle structure of the back. Use a chopping, slashing movement along the back and hip muscles and spine. This is good for easing muscle fatigue (Fig. 3–29).

VIBRATING THE EARS

The index finger is inserted into one ear at a time and vibrated slowly to relax the patient who has nervous tension and general fatigue (Fig. 3–30).

**FIG. 3–23
USING THE ELBOW**

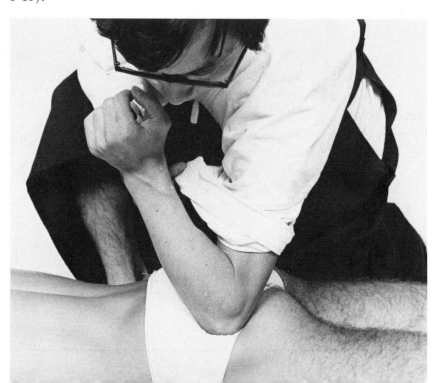

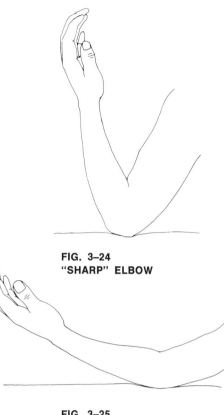

FIG. 3–24
"SHARP" ELBOW

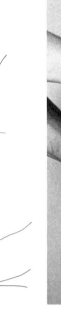

FIG. 3–25
RELAXED ELBOW

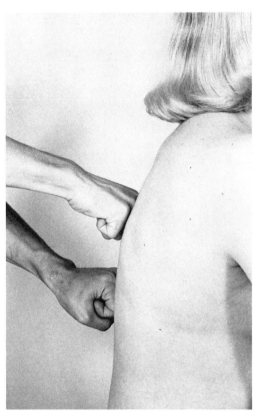

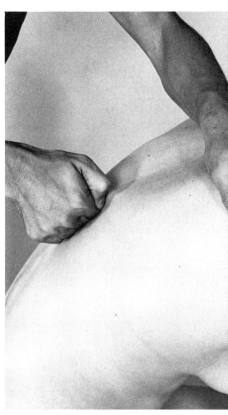

FIGS. 3–26 AND 3–27   USING FIST ALONG THE SPINE

FIG. 3–28   PULLING THE BACK MUSCLES   FIG. 3–29   KNIFE TECHNIQUE   FIG. 3–30   VIBRATING THE EARS

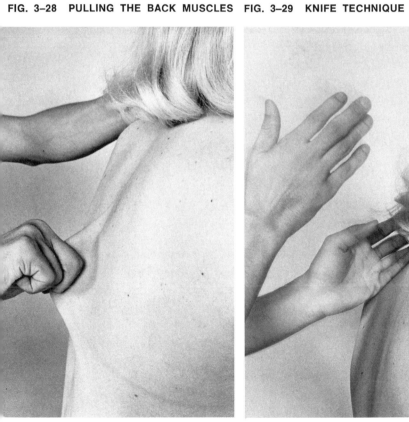

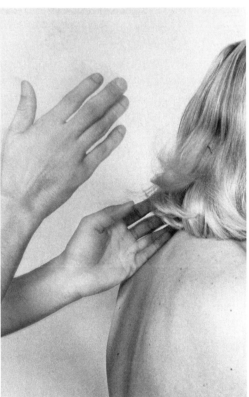

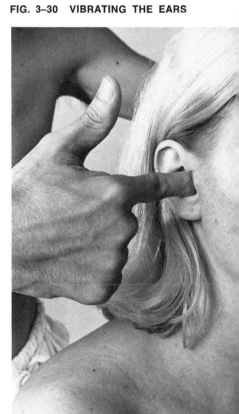

4. Back Shiatsu

A strong, flexible back is absolutely essential to health and a feeling of comfort and well-being. Yet, the back, like the neck, is one of the first places to store tension, resulting in muscle pain and stiffness. In America, where it is so easy for our backs to become weak and tense from lack of exercise, backache is a common ailment. Although you can and must exercise to keep your back healthy (see suggested exercises in chapter 10), you cannot reach your own back to Shiatsu it when it feels uncomfortable. So you must depend on the skill and availability of someone else's fingers to keep energy flowing in one of the most important areas of your body.

I like to call the back the "mirror" of the body because it reflects malfunctions of major organs in the Associated Points in the Bladder Meridian, which runs in a straight line on both sides of the spine. These points (*yu* in Japanese) are connected to the major organs in a way we cannot yet confidently explain, which is why we call them "Associated Points"— they are associated with organs. When you apply pressure on the Associated Points, an abnormal degree of pain and stiffness may indicate a malfunction in the liver, kidney, heart, or other organs. Of course, you cannot rely completely on back diagnosis, since the pain can be caused by structural, muscular, or posture problems. You must check other points, such as the Alarm Points, related to the organ in question and diagnose the *Hara* (or abdominal area) (see chapter 5) before you can get even an indication that something is wrong .

Associated Points in the Bladder Meridian

In Oriental medicine, especially in Shiatsu, diagnosis and treatment are both accomplished in the same way. So, when we find and press the Associated Points on the back, we are treating as well as diagnosing an ailment in the corresponding organ.

As you know, the first Bladder Meridian is located between the "transverse processes" of the spine on both sides—that is, between the vertebrae and the bones which extend to the side of each vertebra. Yon can find the first thoracic vertebra by bending the patient's head forward and looking for the large knobby vertebra at the end of the neck, which is the seventh cervical vertebra. The next vertebra down is the first thoracic vertebra. If two large knobs surface and you can't tell which belongs to the neck, slowly rotate the patient's head. The vertebra that moves with the neck is the seventh cervical. So the first Bladder Meridian point on the back, Bladder #11, is located between the first two thoracic vertebrae; Bladder #12 is between the second and third, and so forth. You may also have trouble distinguishing the lumbar from the thoracic vertebrae. The navel is located in the same place as the point between the second and third lumbar vertebrae. If you wrap a string around the body so it passes across the navel, it will also pass between the second and third lumbar vertebrae on the back. You can find the fifth and sixth thoracic vertebrae by tying a string around the chest across the nipple line. If your patient is a large-breasted woman, have her lie on the floor in order to find the true nipple line.

Following is a list of the Associated Points on the Bladder Meridian, the organs to which they correspond, their locations, and the problems that can be treated by pressing them.

Japanese Name	English Name	Organ	Location	Problem
Hai Yu	BL #13	lung	3–4T	cold, asthma, bronchitis
Ketsu Yin Yu	BL #14	heart constrictor	4–5T	hypertension, palpitations
Shin Yu	BL #15	heart	5–6T	heart-related problems
Kan Yu	BL #18	liver	9–10T	liver problems
Tan Yu	BL #19	gall bladder	10–11T	gall bladder malfunctions
Hi Yu	BL #20	spleen (pancreas)	11–12T	pancreas malfunctions
I Yu	BL #21	stomach	12T–1L	stomach malfunctions
San Shyo Yu	BL #22	triple heater	1–2L	circulation problems
Jin Yu	BL #23	kidney	2–3L	This point is the "center of energy." Treat to revitalize entire body. Also kidney malfunctions
Dai Cho Yu	BL #25	large intestine	4–5L	constipation and large intestine malfunctions
Sho Cho Yu	BL #27	small intestine	1st indentation in sacrum	small intestine malfunctions
Bo Ko Yu	BL #28	bladder	2nd indentation in sacrum	bladder malfunctions

Key: T—Thoracic vertebra; L—Lumbar vertebra; —"between"

65

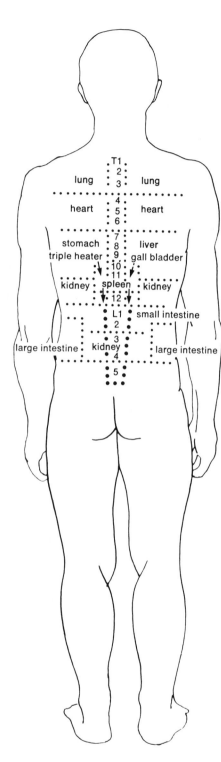

The following labels appear on the figure:

T1, 2, 3 — lung, lung
4, 5, 6 — heart, heart
7, 8, 9 — stomach, triple heater, liver, gall bladder
10, 11 — kidney, spleen, kidney
12 —
L1, 2, 3, 4 — small intestine, large intestine, kidney, large intestine
5

Map of Back Pain

As you are pressing the Associated Points you will often find the patient's stiffness or discomfort cannot be pinned down to one specific point. A problematic organ will sometimes affect a more general area of the back. Fig. 4–1 is a "Map of the Back" which shows the relationship of the vertebrae and surrounding areas to specific organs.

Other Ways to Diagnose the Back

The first way to diagnose a patient by looking at the back is to observe the muscles on both sides of the spine. A healthy person's spine is sunk deep in the center of the longitudinal muscles. An unhealthy person's spine may have vertebrae that are easy to count. An unhealthy back may also have muscles that are not equally balanced on both sides, so that the patient carries his weight more to one side than the other. If you find curvature of the spinal vertebrae, or a big lump or curve in the muscles, there may be a problem in an organ or bodily function corresponding to that area of the back. Prominent muscles on the right side of the center back may indicate liver problems or gallstones. Prominent muscles on the left side may indicate stomach problems. Heart problems, especially in the valves, can appear in the form of painful stiffness on the left side of the back, just below the shoulder blade. We cannot be completely sure if the pain and stiffness appear because the organ is in trouble; or if the pain and stiffness, created by poor posture and lack of exercise, lead to a malfunction of the associated organ.

PALM DIAGNOSIS

Have the patient lie on his stomach and place your palm vertically on his spine. Starting at the top of the spine and working your way down, press gently. You will be able to tell where there is stiffness or spasm. Backache, shoulder pain, stomach ache, and hiccups can be alleviated with this technique as well.

SLIDING DIAGNOSIS

Have the patient bend forward so his spinal column is accentuated. Take your index and middle fingers and slide them firmly down the spine from the neck (if you are standing behind the patient), or up the spine if you are standing in front of him (Fig. 4–2). Bumps, bulges, or stiffness indicate a problem in the corresponding organ.

SCRATCH TECHNIQUE

The patient lies in a relaxed position on his stomach. With the thumbnails of both hands scratch along both sides of the spine from top to bottom. You will observe red lines on both sides. If the line is broken or discontinued in any area, the organ corresponding to that area may be malfunctioning.

Precaution: Remember that these are only preliminary tests. Stiffness or pain *may* indicate an organ malfunction, but not necessarily. Don't try to

**FIG. 4–2
SLIDING DIAGNOSIS
OF THE BACK**

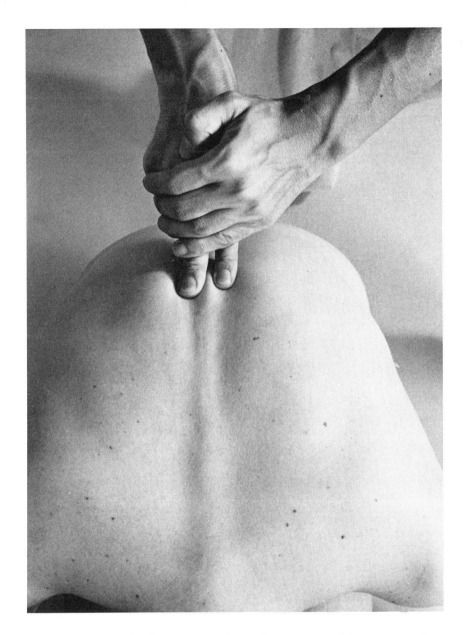

cure any suspected ailments yourself with Shiatsu, or diagnose a patient without professional help.

How to Give Back Shiatsu

Before giving back Shiatsu review the Shiatsu techniques in chapter 3, many of which are applied to the back. Before applying pressure to the tsubo on the Bladder Meridian lines with your thumbs, you will want to loosen and relax the muscles of the patient's back and stretch the spine, all of which will make your treatment of the tsubos more effective.

STRETCHING THE BACK

The patient lies on his stomach. Place the palm of one hand on the upper back and the palm of the other on the sacrum. Using your body

**FIG. 4–3
STRETCHING THE BACK**

**FIG. 4–4
CROSSING THE ARMS
AND STRETCHING
THE BACK**

weight for pressure and keeping your elbows straight, stretch the upper back toward the head and the sacrum toward the feet (Fig. 4–3). If you have especially long arms, cross them to get a better stretch (Fig. 4–4).

Now stretch the spine by pressing with the heel of your hand between the vertebrae. Bend the patient's legs with your other hand and stretch by pressing upward as the patient exhales (Fig. 4–5). If you need stronger

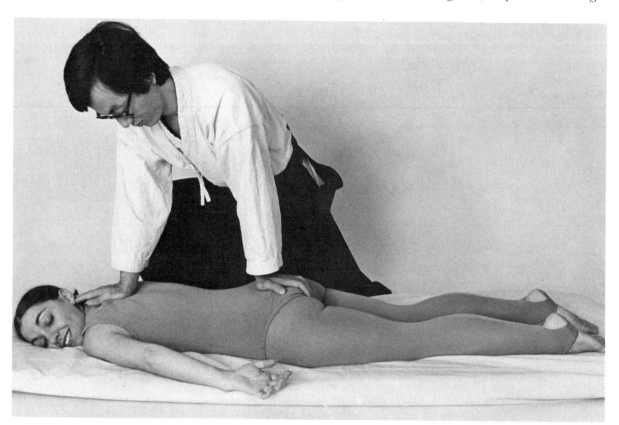

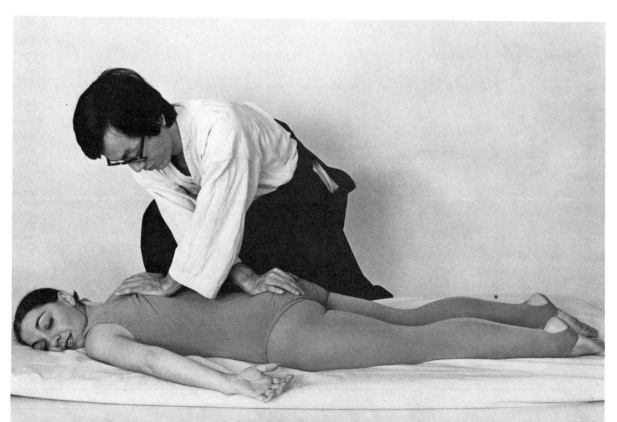

pressure you can use your foot on the patient's back in much the same fashion. The space between his vertebrae should fall between the first two toes of your foot. Hold his legs in a bent position and step down as he exhales (Fig. 4–6). If the patient is weak, old, has fragile bones, or has been taking large doses of cortisone (which weakens the bones), or if you are heavy yourself, don't use these techniques.

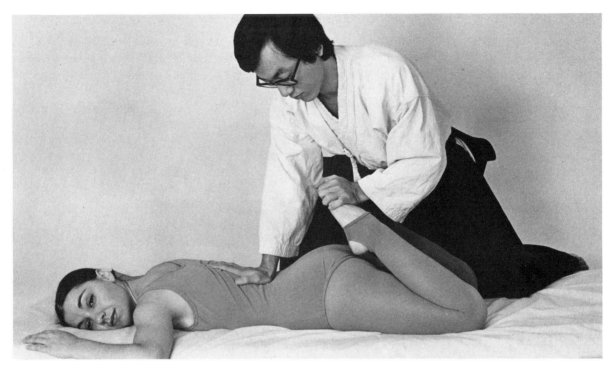

FIG. 4–5
STRETCHING THE
SPINAL PROCESS
WITH THE HEEL
OF THE HAND

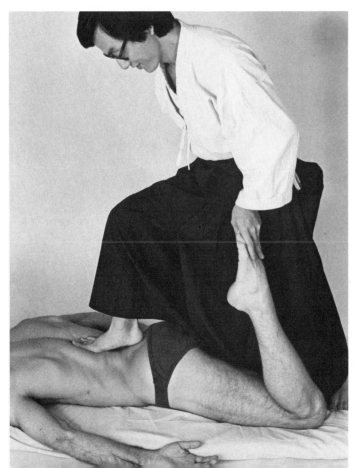

FIG. 4–6
STRETCHING WITH
THE FOOT

SQUEEZING THE MUSCLES ALONG THE TORSO

Interlock your fingers, and with the palms down squeeze the back upward along the sides of the torso (Fig. 4–7). If the patient's muscles are especially tight, bend his legs back to help you distinguish the muscles along the spine. Squeeze upward again (Fig. 4–8). This technique is good for lower-back ache and general fatigue.

ROCKING TECHNIQUE

The patient lies on his side with his top leg in a bent position and his bottom leg straight. If he is on his left side his right arm is relaxed behind him, and vice versa. You can stand, or kneel on one knee. (In Fig. 4–9

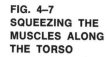

**FIG. 4–7
SQUEEZING THE
MUSCLES ALONG
THE TORSO**

**FIG. 4–8
BENDING LEGS
AND SQUEEZING**

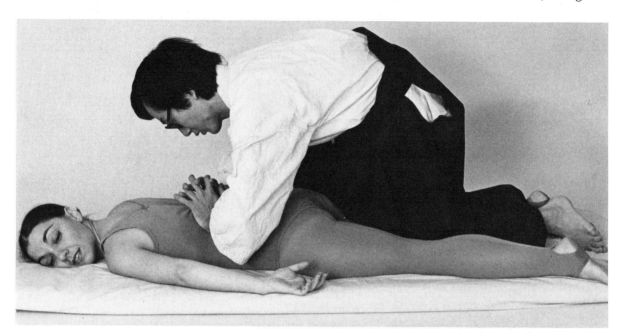

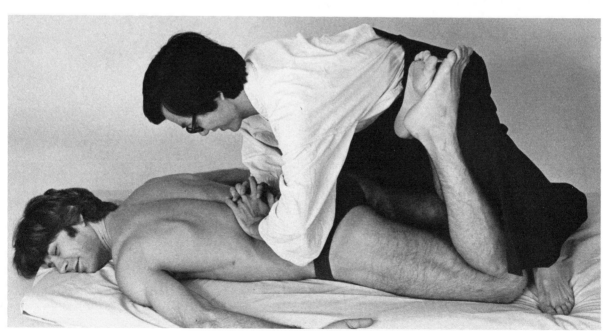

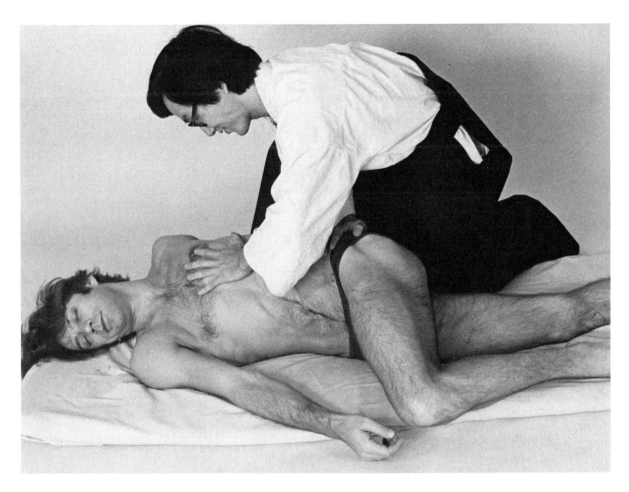

FIG. 4–9
ROCKING TECHNIQUE

the patient is lying on his right side, and I have my left hand on his chest and my right hand on his hip.) Using a rocking motion, push his chest toward his left shoulder and his hip toward his navel. This helps to loosen the back and relieve backache.

SLASHING THE SHOULDER BLADE

Relax the patient's shoulder and then, using the blade of your hand in a slashing manner, place your hand into the groove between the shoulder blade and the back. Using your other hand for pressure, manipulate the muscle back and forth for three to five minutes. This is good for frozen shoulder, difficulty in moving the arm, backache, and nervous tension (Fig. 4–10, see p. 72).

APPLYING PRESSURE TO THE TSUBOS

The basic procedure for giving back Shiatsu is to apply pressure with your thumbs to the tsubos on the first and second Bladder Meridians, which are located on both sides of the spine (see illustrations in chapter 2). Earlier in this chapter I explained how to find the tsubos on the first Bladder Meridian and the Associated Points. The second Bladder Meridian is located about three inches from each side of the spine, just off the long muscles that run down the back. Remember, when applying pressure:

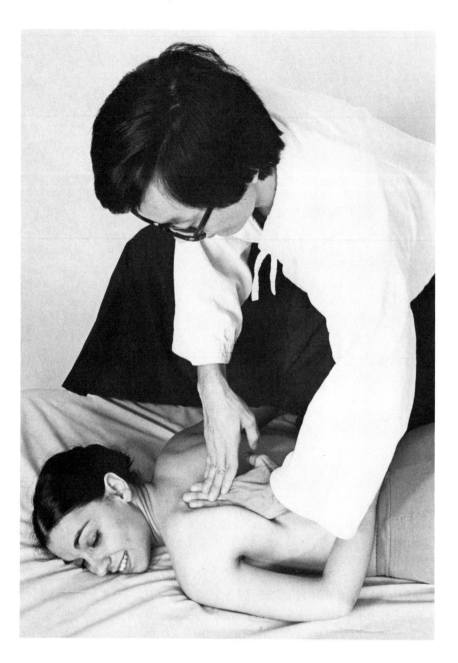

**FIG. 4-10
SLASHING THE
SHOULDER BLADE**

1. Stretch both arms. If you bend your elbows you get tired easily and cannot give enough pressure.

2. Come as close to the patient as possible in order to use your weight most effectively.

3. Relax the patient. To give Shiatsu is to give love and joy—not pain.

4. Press straight down at a 90-degree angle.

VIBRATION TECHNIQUE

While pressing you can vibrate your thumb very subtly. This makes the patient feel more comfortable and relaxed. Fig. 4-11 shows the proper way to give Shiatsu to the points on the first Bladder Meridian. If you need more pressure, put one thumb on top of the other. Press each tsubo for five to seven seconds, three times. Again, make sure you press as he exhales. If the patient feels too sensitive to the pressure, you can alleviate his pain by continuously vibrating the palm of one hand on his back while you give pressure with the other (Fig. 4–12).

PRESSING KAN GEN YU (BLADDER #26)

Bladder #26 is a very important tsubo because it is in a joint. Treatment of Bladder #26 can help lower-back ache, tired legs, digestive and sexual problems. It is located between the fifth lumbar vertebra and the pelvic bone. If you have trouble finding it, bend the patient's knees toward his back, which will make Bladder #26 appear more clearly. Instead of pressing straight down at a 90-degree angle, press in, then upward toward the head for five to seven seconds, three times (see Fig. 3–2).

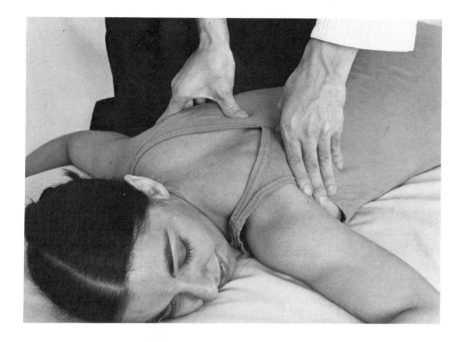

FIG. 4–11
APPLYING PRESSURE
TO THE TSUBO
ON THE FIRST
BLADDER MERIDIAN

FIG. 4–12
VIBRATING THE PALM
WHILE PRESSING THE
TSUBO

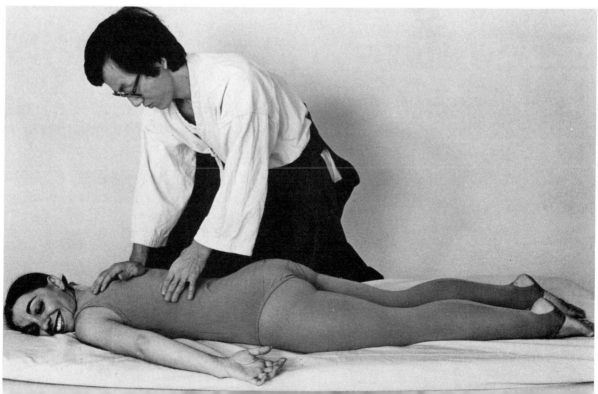

5. Ampuku Therapy

The Hara

Orientals believe that the center of the body's strength is located in the abdominal area, which they call the *Hara*. The Hara, in Western anatomical terms, is the area between the rib cage and the pelvic bone which contains most of our vital organs and where the digestive and reproductive functions take place. Since food is digested in this area and we receive our bodily energy from food, if the Hara is not functioning well, we cannot use food energy to produce life-maintaining or self-healing power.

I love plants. I have many plants in my school and office. Sometimes I find that even if a plant has a profusion of leaves and looks healthy, it dies anyway. I wonder why. I often find that it had rotten, dead roots. In a human being the Hara is the root. If your Hara is rotten you are chronically weak and get sick easily. You must cultivate the Hara, like a plant, to gain health so you can lead an active, vigorous life. For the Shiatsu therapist the Hara is the most important part of the body. In Japan there are "Hara specialists" who work only on this part of the body. This type of Shiatsu is called Ampuku therapy.

In the Caucasus area of Russia there are people who live to a ripe old age of one hundred years, sometimes more. These people massage themselves every morning with a dry cloth or leaves—a practice very similar to Ampuku. This is one of the reasons they are so healthy and live so long. In Japan everyone is aware of the importance of the Hara. The Japanese language, with its dozens of idiomatic expressions referring to the Hara, reflects this attitude. For example, *Hara guroi*, literally translated "dirty Hara," is an expression used to describe a cunning, sneaky, or dishonest person; *Hara o tateru*, literally meaning "upset Hara," describes an angry or upset person; *Hara ga aru*, meaning "to have Hara," describes a brave person with energy and spirit; and of course you are familiar with the term *Hara kiri*, meaning to "cut off the Hara," a ritual form of suicide in which the Hara is cut with a knife. (Less literally, *Hara kiri* describes a person willing to take responsibility for his own actions.)

I've found that people who live in modern societies pay little or no attention to this most important center of energy production. There are several routine experiments you can do to demonstrate to yourself the importance of the Hara. If you are a dog owner, rub or gently press your dog's stomach when he is lying on his back. He will enjoy this so much he may fall asleep. If your baby is crying, feeling flustered or uncomfortable, put your hands on the stomach and sing a lullaby. He or she will love it. When you are really upset, all your tension is concentrated in the Hara. Touch it next time you are anxious and you will see that this is true. When a Japanese person gets angry, he squeezes his Hara, both to express his fury and to relieve it at the same time. Try this yourself. Relaxing softens the Hara and simultaneously relieves the emotional condition that caused it to become so tense to begin with. Zen monks, who are instructed to keep their minds on the breathing in the Hara to help them attain the state of *Mu* (or "no mind"), relax the Hara by placing their palms on the area and rubbing in a circle sixty times. Try this the next time you are upset.

The Hara and Movement

In the traditional Japanese Noh dance, the dancer must move his body from the Hara. Each movement, no matter which part of the body is involved, must begin in the Hara area. This is also true for other forms of dance. Even in normal activities if your gravity is not created in the Hara you will lose your balance easily.

The type of boxer known as the "dancer" also relies on the Hara, as the Hara controls leg movement. He fights defensively and aggressively, dodging and blocking as he moves around the floor looking for the correct moment to corner his opponent. The other kind of boxer, the "slugger," relies on his strength and punching technique. He stops the "dancer" by constantly delivering heavy blows to the Hara.

The Hara and Sex

The part of the Hara which is the storage place of all our energy is called the *Tan Den*. To find the Tan Den place the palm of your hand, with the thumb folded under, on your stomach with the forefinger just below your navel. The Tan Den is just below the place where your ring finger is lying. It is sometimes called *Ki Kai* or Conception Vessel #6. The Tan Den produces all of our vital force, including sexual desire. People who don't have a happy sex life have problems with the Tan Den area. To cure sexual problems such as impotence, premature ejaculation, frigidity, and absence of orgasm you should have Tan Den Ampuku every day. Later in this chapter I will describe exactly how this is done.

Ampuku Diagnosis

In the old days Oriental people did not have x-ray machines to view the inner workings of the body. The only equipment they used to discover what was happening in the abdomen was the palm and fingers. All diagnosis was done through touch. Since the Hara is the center of all our energy (known as *Ki* in Japanese and *Chi* in Chinese), it is the barometer for the rest of the body. You may look fine, but if you have a "dead Hara" you are unhealthy. You may be ill, but if you have a healthy Hara, you are basically "in good condition" and will recover quickly. In my career I have often found that a patient with an unhealthy Hara is not easy to cure and must be warned to have patience.

To diagnose the Hara ask the patient to lie on his back and bend his legs so the hara is relaxed. If he is uncomfortable you can use a stool or pillows to support his bent legs. Ask him to breathe with his mouth open, which will help him to relax. First examine the surface of the abdomen. If the navel is in the center of the body and is slender and deep, it indicates the patient is healthy. A large, shallow navel can be, generally speaking, an indication of poor health. (A navel which "sticks out" in a child will recede in a healthy adult.) A Hara is healthy when the lower Hara (below the navel) is more muscular, more flexible, and juts out a little more than the upper Hara (above the navel). If the skin color is abnormally red, dark, or pale, this may indicate an unhealthy Hara.

For a general diagnosis of the internal Hara, place your relaxed hand on the abdomen and move it around gently. Don't press. Feel for stiffness in the abdominal region and listen for gurgling sounds, moving gas, and test for high temperature, sweating, or dryness—all signs of problems (Fig. 5–1). In the photograph the patient's legs are straight. As she bends her legs I can touch more deeply and precisely for a more effective diagnosis.

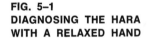
**FIG. 5–1
DIAGNOSING THE HARA
WITH A RELAXED HAND**

Now check the internal organs. In general, what you are looking for is stiffness and resistance in the stomach and liver, which may indicate prob-

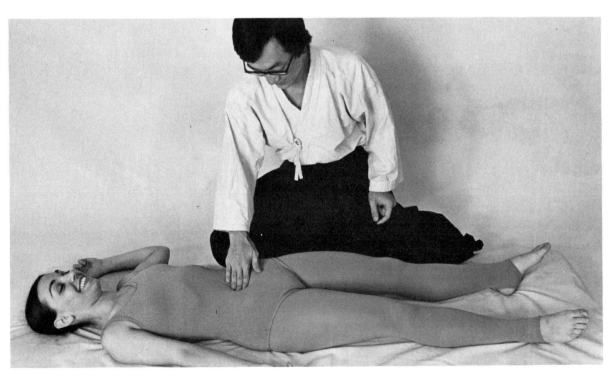

lems in these organs. The stomach is on the left side of the Hara and the liver on the right (see Fig. 5–2). To check the stomach put your relaxed hand on the left side of the Hara. When the patient exhales, slide your fingers up slowly under the rib cage. Slide in, don't press down. If you cannot slide your fingers beneath the rib cage, or if there is stiffness and pain, there may be stomach problems such as ulcers or malfunctions of the digestive tract. Continue to slide your fingers deeper into the rib cage and watch for signs of pain or stiffness (Figs. 5–3 and 5–4). The liver is checked in the same way, only the thumbs or fingers are slid up under the *right* rib cage (Fig. 5–5). If you cannot do this or hit a stiff or resistant

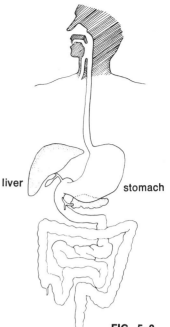

FIG. 5–2
AN INTERNAL VIEW
OF THE HARA AREA

FIG. 5–3
SLIDING THE FINGERS
UNDER THE LEFT RIB CAGE
TO CHECK THE STOMACH

FIG. 5–4
SLIDING THE FINGERS
IN DEEPER

FIG. 5–5
CHECKING THE LIVER

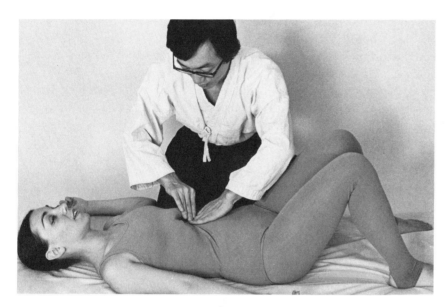

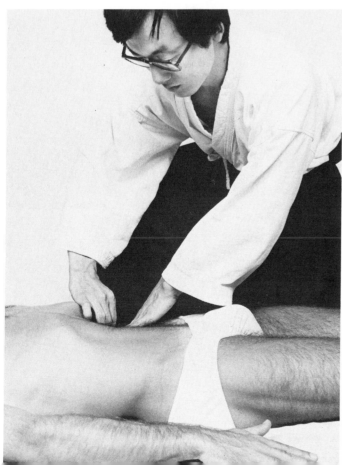

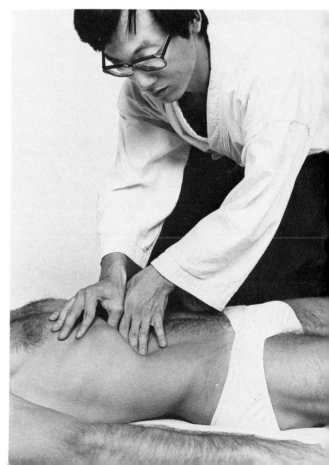

area the patient may have a liver problem. If he is a big drinker, gets little sleep, works too hard, and has diarrhea or constipation, he could well have a swollen liver. You can diagnose your own stomach and liver by lying on your back, bending your knees with the soles of your feet placed on the floor, then sliding your fingers up under both sides of the rib cage.

Compare both sides of your patient's (or your own) abdomen. Tension and stiffness along the right side could mean the patient is suffering not only from liver trouble, but from headache, shoulder pain, dizziness, or insomnia. Tension on the left side might mean diarrhea, constipation, or poor circulation. If you hear the sound of sloshing water as you massage, the patient has digestive troubles. Bubbling in the stomach means a stomach is functioning weakly. A swollen or hanging stomach is not healthy either. If the gas expelled from the body smells bad or if there is chronic bad breath, digestive problems may be the cause. When you check your own Hara, the sound of moving water before or long after your last meal may tell you about weak digestion, diarrhea, or gastritis. Before you get diarrhea you may feel something "working" in your Hara and hear thunderous gas noises as well. (Don't be confused by the gas sounds that mean you are hungry.)

Detecting Stomach Cancer

**FIG. 5–6
GIVING AMPUKU—FOUR
FINGER TECHNIQUE**

Stomach cancer kills many thousands of Japanese every year and in 1974 the American Cancer Society estimated that 14,700 Americans died

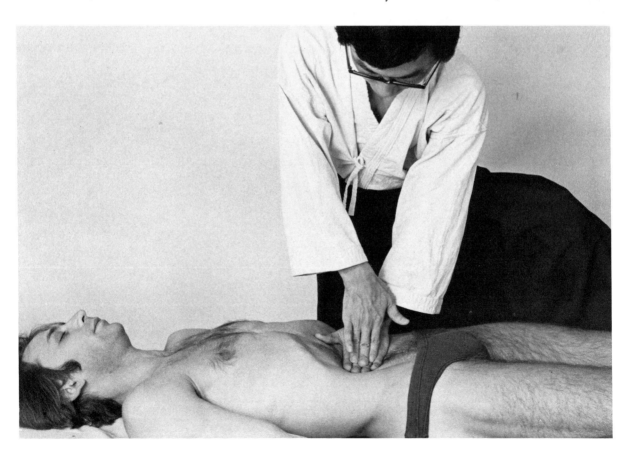

78

of it. One of the main reasons, says the ACS, is a superfluity of refined starch and not enough fresh fruits and vegetables in the diet. Ampuku diagnosis can sometimes help detect stomach cancer. Make sure the patient has not eaten recently. Bend his legs while he relaxes on his back and touch his stomach, looking for hard, lumpy tissue (some call it "cauliflower" in the stomach). If you find the "cauliflower" while you press hard, and there is no pain, you can suspect an ulcer or stomach cancer and send the patient immediately for professional diagnosis and treatment. Do not confuse "cauliflower" with stomach gas, which also feels hard at times.

Ampuku Pulse Diagnosis

Have the patient lie on his back as before, bend his legs, and relax his mouth. Sit to his left side, placing both of your stretched hands on the left side of the navel where the artery runs, about an inch or two away from the navel. Press gently inward and check for a strong pulse. If it is so strong that you feel it in your shoulders, the person is sick, perhaps from bad digestion, diarrhea, constipation, or ulcers. Make sure the patient has not eaten for at least two hours before diagnosis and rests at least a half hour beforehand.

How to Give Ampuku Therapy

We give Ampuku therapy for general well-being, good digestion, relaxation, and a more satisfying sex life. When giving Ampuku we never press a specific point, or tsubo. Instead we press a more generalized area of the abdomen gently and slowly while the patient exhales. Here are some of the techniques we use in giving Ampuku:

1. FOUR-FINGER TECHNIQUE

Have the patient lie on his back, relax the Hara, and preferably bend his legs. Relax your fingers. Place the fingers of one hand over those of the other, for a more concentrated force. Start pressing just below the solar plexus and continue along the edge of the rib cage, tracing the abdomen down to the hipbone and to the pelvic bone. Then continue in a clockwise direction up the other side of the abdomen. Increase the pressure slowly and push only when the patient is exhaling. Never press the solar plexus or the navel. Complete the circle three times (Fig. 5–6).

2. THREE-FINGER TECHNIQUE

Follow the four-finger procedure, but use three fingers. Do this three times.

3. TWO-FINGER TECHNIQUE

Follow the same procedure using two fingers. With two fingers you can increase the amount of pressure slightly, and press a little deeper. Be very gentle. Again, three times.

4. ONE-THUMB TECHNIQUE

Place one thumb on top of the other. Increase the amount of pressure gradually, pressing deeper and longer. Again, begin below the solar plexus and continue clockwise in a circle three times (Fig. 5–7).

You may use all of these techniques or only one or alternate them, again depending on your perception of the effect they are having on your patient.

5. PINCHING THE MUSCLES

Pick up the muscles along the patient's side and pinch them with your entire hand toward the outside of his body. Pinch as he exhales, three to five times. Don't pinch the intestine. This is good for tired legs and backache (Fig. 5–8).

FIG. 5–7
THUMB TECHNIQUE

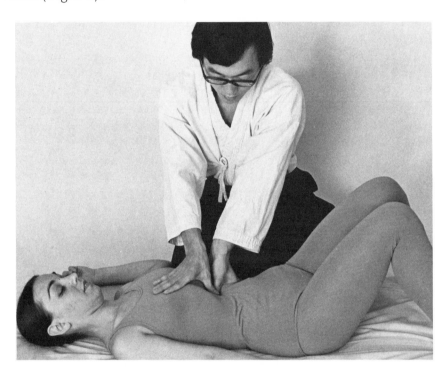

FIG. 5–8
PINCHING THE MUSCLES

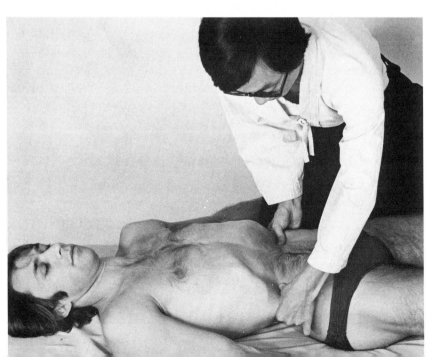

6. LIFTING THE HARA

Place your hands on the muscles along the patient's spine and lift him up slowly from underneath while he is exhaling, vibrating your hands at the same time. This is good for tired legs and the lower back (Fig. 5–9).

7. SQUEEZING THE ABDOMINAL AREA

Gently squeeze the abdominal area up and release it, making sure the fingers are loose and relaxed. Do this vertically and horizontally, twenty times a session. This is good therapy for constipation, all digestive problems, tension, and sexual problems (Fig. 5–10).

8. ROCKING THE HARA

Place one hand on top of the other and put them on the side of the

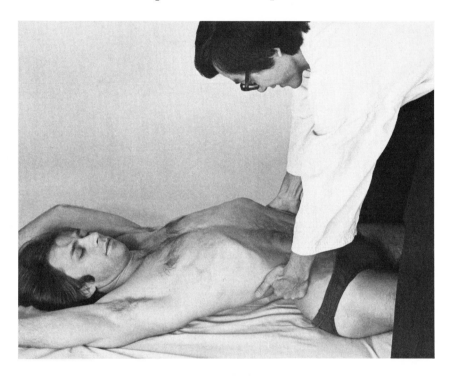

FIG. 5–9
LIFTING THE HARA

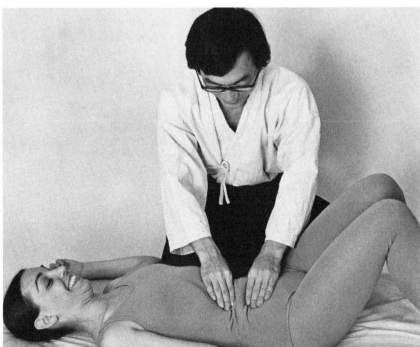

FIG. 5–10
SQUEEZING THE
ABDOMINAL AREA

Hara. When the patient exhales, pull the abdomen toward your body, then press back toward the patient's body, rocking back and forth. Don't press hard. Good for digestive problems and insomnia (Fig. 5–11).

9. TWISTING THE BODY

Put a relaxed open hand on the patient's rib cage. Have him bend the top knee and place that leg on top of the bottom leg (as in the picture). Then "twist" the patient's body by pushing the bent leg toward you, creating a stretch in the patient's abdominal area. Don't press the rib cage, just rest your hand on it for leverage. Do this five or seven times. Good for abdominal muscle spasms (Fig. 5–12).

Tan Den Ampuku

Regular Tan Den Ampuku cures sexual problems and stimulates life energy. To begin with, give the patient a rubdown and Shiatsu for ten minutes on the loins, where the legs meet the torso (Fig. 5–13). Then find the Tan Den tsubo, or Conception Vessel #4, which is four fingers below the navel (as described earlier in this chapter), just over the small intestine. By touching this vessel a therapist can judge the quality of your sex life. If your sexual energies are in good working order, the Tan Den is soft but flexible. Shiatsu is given here for about ten minutes. Press the

**FIG. 5–11
ROCKING THE HARA**

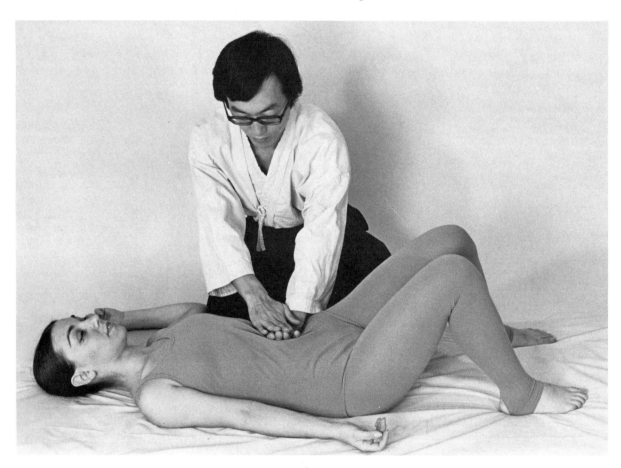

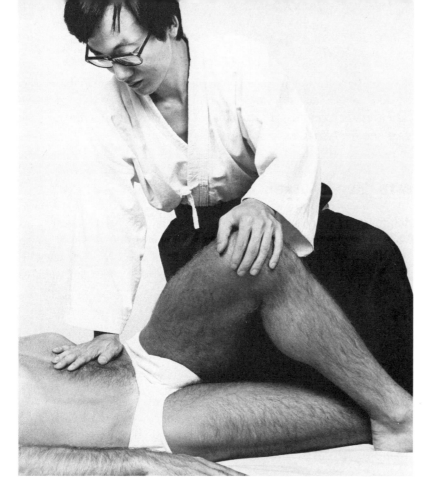

FIG. 5–12
TWISTING THE BODY

FIG. 5–13
RUBBING THE LOINS

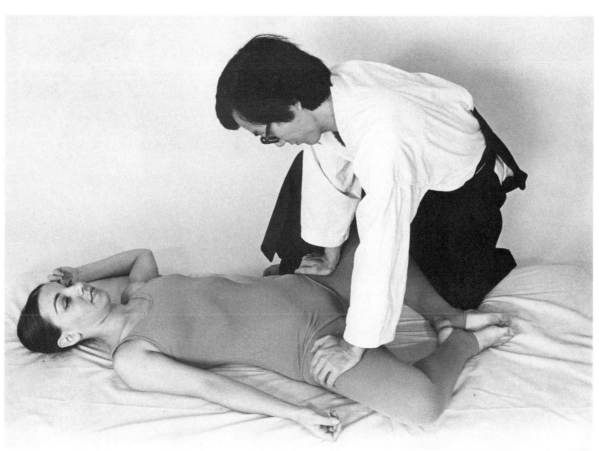

Tan Den tsubo with the palm of your hand and release. Continue this procedure, going "deeper" and applying more pressure with each exhalation of the patient. The patient will actually be able to feel the energy gathering from deep inside.

How to Give Yourself Ampuku

Often there is no one to give you Shiatsu when you need it most. This shouldn't prevent you from keeping the Hara area in good condition on your own. There are several Ampuku treatments you can give yourself, which will aid general health, digestion, and help you to relax and achieve a tranquil state of mind.

**FIG. 5–14
SELF-AMPUKU**

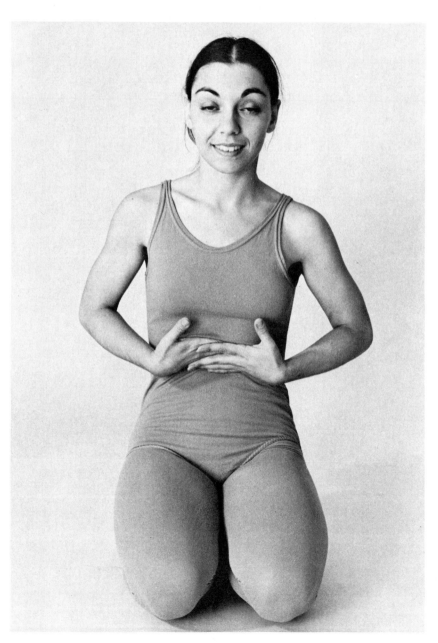

1. Sit on your knees, relaxing your abdomen. Clasp your hands on the Hara and breathe in. As you exhale, press your hands deeply into the Hara. Bend forward for deeper penetration (Fig. 5–14). Start on the stomach area and proceed downward toward the pelvic bone, then around in a clockwise direction. Do this for about five minutes.

2. With one hand on top of the other and your palms on the navel, rotate in a clockwise direction sixty times.

3. Interlock your fingers and squeeze the Hara while exhaling.

4. Lie on your back, bend your legs, relax the Hara, and open your mouth. Place both hands just below the solar plexus and press gently. Then move on to the stomach, navel, and Tan Den area, pressing in a clockwise direction. Rub down and stroke, rotating the Hara.

5. Placing four fingers on the Hara, press lightly around in a clockwise direction. Then follow the same procedure with three fingers, two fingers, and the thumb, as you did to your patient.

6. With your palm push the Hara to one side and pull back with the fingertips.

7. Place one hand on top of the other on the navel area and vibrate the hands gently, moving them in an up-and-down motion.

Any of these exercises is good to do before you eat, and as soon as you wake up, before getting out of bed. If you feel gas during the exercises, let it out.

Redistributing Your Weight with Ampuku

The abdomen is the easiest place to gain weight and the easiest place to lose it, too. While you are dieting you can redistribute the fat around your midsection by pinching the fatty area back and forth and then up and down. Do this squeezing procedure for twenty or thirty minutes daily, while you are sitting at your desk or watching television. Do not worry if you feel a pinching pain—this means you are doing it correctly. Actually, you are not eliminating extra fat, but spreading it out so that it bulges less under clothing.

6. Neck Shiatsu

Pain in the Neck?

Neck Shiatsu is very important because so many of us have pains in our necks. Why? In order to sustain these heavy heads of ours, the muscles of the neck must work extremely hard and often become tired and stiff. Unless the spine is completely straight, the neck does not have the support of a strong line of vertebrae and has to carry more of the weight of the head by itself. Most of our spines curve one way or another; in fact, only about one out of every hundred people has a perfectly straight spine. When the head is carried too far to the right or left, it seems much heavier and the neck has to do double duty. Neck problems can also begin in the legs or lower back. Bad posture of any kind causes tension in the neck. High heels, in fashion with men as well as women nowadays, force the hipbone forward, the lumbar and thoracic vertebrae to curve forward and then back again, and the neck to jut forward—the result is a pretzel-shaped spine and pain in the neck! Also, many meridian lines pass through the neck, which makes it easy for ki-energy to stagnate there. Blockage of ki-energy in the Conception Vessel, Triple Heater, Gall Bladder Governing Vessel, Stomach, and Bladder Meridians, all of which pass through the neck, can cause neck pain and stiffness.

We can help cure nervous tension, headache, shoulder pain, lower-back ache, insomnia, and hypertension with neck Shiatsu. Yet the neck is, without question, the most difficult part of the body to treat with Shiatsu and demands a great deal of skill. I can tell immediately whether a Shiatsu therapist is good or not, and even how long he has been doing Shiatsu, by taking neck Shiatsu from him. One well-known Shiatsu therapist claims it takes three years to master working on the back and legs, but eight years to master the neck.

Why is it so difficult to work on the neck? First of all, the neck is slender, the narrowest part of the body. Since it presents such a small area for your fingers, and the neck tsubos are grouped so closely together, your work must be very precise. Second, many important nerves come and go through the neck, which make it extremely sensitive. Third, the cervical vertebrae can move close to the surface of the body and get easily dislocated by impact. In Western movies we often see the cowboy knock out his opponent by hitting the back of his neck with a gun butt. That is why we cannot press too suddenly or too hard when working on the neck. If you press hard and shock the cervical vertebrae you can damage or dislocate them.

Neck Diagnosis

The neck is the mirror of the body's health. Abnormal pain or stiffness in the neck indicates an unhealthy body and a need for neck Shiatsu.

To diagnose the neck first observe its length and shape. A short, stocky neck, which the Japanese call "wild pig neck," may indicate a Yang-type person with a possible tendency for hypertension and high blood pressure. A long and slender neck ("crane neck" in Japanese) generally indicates a Yin-type person with a possible tendency for lung problems or bronchitis.

Next, rotate the neck in order to test its flexibility. See how far the patient can bend his neck forward and to the sides. Ask him whether it pains him to do this. A healthy neck is relaxed and has a good deal of mobility.

Then touch the neck and feel for stiffness, abnormal tightness, or tension. The patient with nervous tension or hypertension will have a tight, stiff neck; the tighter and stiffer, the unhealthier the patient.

Check the patient's posture. If his spine curves to the right, he will feel stiffness in the left side of his lower back, on the right side of the shoulder blade, and on the left side of the neck; and his left leg will be longer than the right leg. If his spine curves to the left, he will feel stiffness on the right side of the lower back, the left side of the shoulder blade, right side of the neck; and the right leg will be longer. Most of us curve to the right or left in varying degrees.

Next, bend the patient's head forward and check the cervical vertebrae with your index and middle fingers. If any of the vertebrae are protruding abnormally or are buried so deep in the neck you cannot find them they are not in their normal location.

Then ask the patient to poke out his tongue. If his tongue extends toward the left, the left side of the neck is tight; if the tongue extends toward the right, the right side is tight. In each case stiff neck muscles are pulling the tongue toward them.

Ohashi's Acupuncture Point

After several years of experience with Shiatsu and Acupuncture, I discovered a new tsubo in the neck which I named "Ohashi's point." Treatment of this tsubo is beneficial for nervous tension and headache.

Ohashi's point is located between the third and fourth cervical vertebrae, one to one and a half inches on either side of the spinal column, almost on the Bladder Meridian. Since it is difficult to find the first cervical vertebra, find the third by counting upward from the seventh; bend the

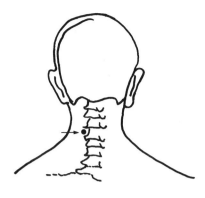

patient's neck forward—the largest protrusion is the seventh cervical vertebra (Fig. 6–1). If you have any doubts about which vertebra belongs to the neck, slowly rotate the patient's head. The large vertebra that turns with the head is the seventh cervical vertebra.

To press Ohashi's point, have the patient lie on his back. You are at one side of his head. Relax his neck muscles by gently bending the head toward the side you are sitting on. Use either the index or middle finger and press in very gently at the point between the third and fourth vertebrae. Then press upward toward the patient's mouth. He will be able to feel sensation along the Bladder Meridian and the back.

How to Give Neck Shiatsu

Here are a variety of techniques for neck Shiatsu which you can develop into a continuous massage.

MOVING FINGERS ON BACK OF NECK

The patient lies on his back. Sit at the patient's head and move the four fingers of both hands around the back of his neck. Make sure your fingers are massaging the *back* of the neck and not the edges or near the throat. Move the fingers of each hand toward one another, not toward the patient's throat. The patient must be relaxed, his mouth open, and his head down. If he has not relaxed, relax the neck yourself by moving and shaking it (Fig. 6–2).

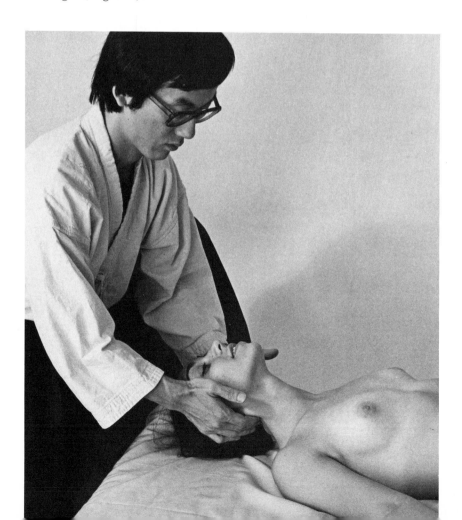

Then do the same thing with three fingers, two fingers, and then the middle or index finger. Press the points along the sides of the back of the neck, including Ohashi's point. This is good for relaxing stiff muscles, nervous tension, insomnia, and headache.

MIDDLE FINGER TECHNIQUE

Place one middle finger over the other middle finger. Press gently in the spaces between the cervical vertebra, upward and in toward the mouth. This technique is good for headache, nervous tension, and fever (Fig. 6–3).

STRETCHING THE CHIN

To help a patient with a stiff neck, lift up his head with your fingers and stretch his chin down toward his chest as far as possible. Advise the patient not to try and help you move his head with his own muscles, but to relax and let you do the work (Fig. 6–4).

**FIG. 6–3
MIDDLE FINGER
TECHNIQUE**

**FIG. 6–4
STRETCHING
THE CHIN**

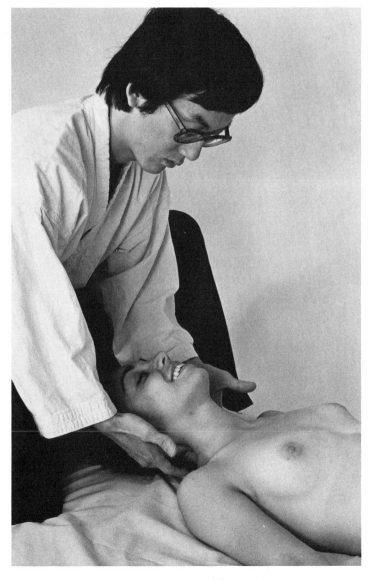

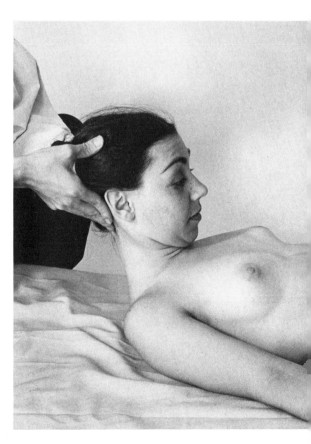

89

PRESSING TSUBOS WITH THE THUMB

The patient is in a sitting position with his back straight. Kneel on one side of him and put one knee into the small of his back for support. Place one hand on the patient's forehead and rest the other hand on the side of his neck. Then press Bladder #10, Gall Bladder #20, and Governing Vessel #15 with the thumb, using the hand you have placed on the patient's forehead to bend his head *toward* the pressure of your thumb. This increases the pressure. Press only when the patient exhales; if he seems to be tensing under the pressure, "fighting back," or if he is extremely uncomfortable, stop!—the technique isn't working. This technique helps headaches and eye problems and relieves the neck aches often caused by colds (Figs. 6–5 and 6–6). In the illustrations I am pressing Bladder #10.

HEADBAND TECHNIQUE

This technique is essentially the same as the one above, except the use of a headband enables you to press tsubos with both thumbs.

Fold a piece of cloth so it is about three inches wide. Holding your hands palms upward, thread it under the little finger, over the three

**FIGS. 6–5 AND 6–6
PRESSING TSUBO
WITH THE THUMB**

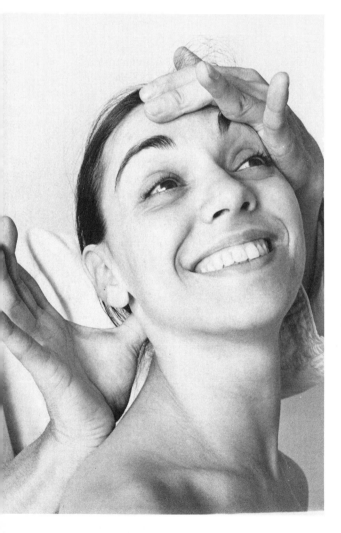
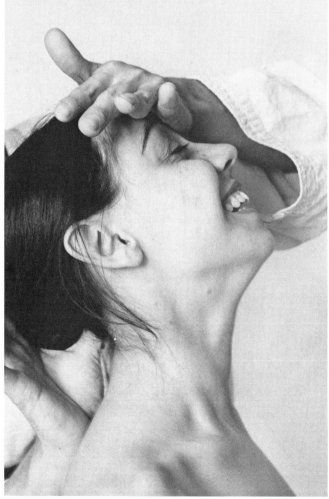

middle fingers, and under the thumb. Then turn your hands over so the backs are on top. Then make a fist. This secures the headband. Place the band around the patient's forehead and with your free thumbs press Bladder #10, Governing Vessel #15, Ohashi's point, and Gall Bladder #20 (Fig. 6–7). Use the headband to pull the patient's head toward the pressure exerted by the thumbs. In the previous technique you used your hand to pull the patient's head toward the pressure of one thumb.

PINCHING THE NECK UPWARD

Take the back of the neck between your fingers and pull upward in a rhythmic motion. This loosens up tension and relaxes muscles. It's also good for lessening the symptoms of fatigue (Fig. 6–8).

**FIG. 6–8
PINCHING THE
NECK UPWARD**

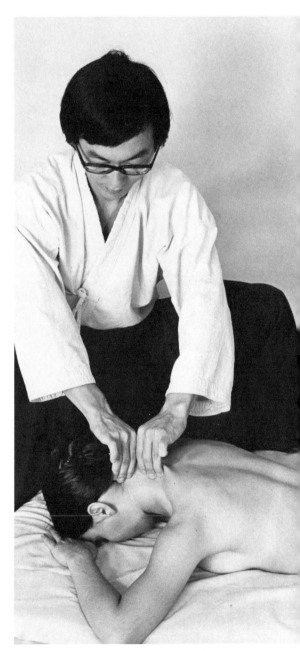

**FIG. 6–7
HEADBAND TECHNIQUE**

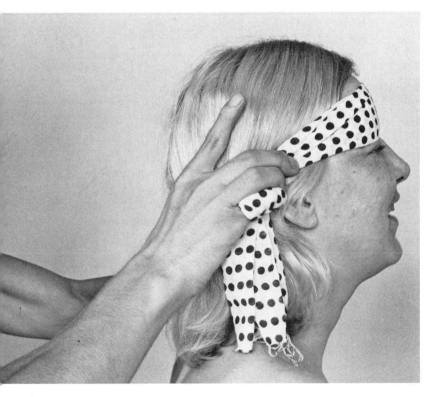

RIDING THE BICYCLE

Sit at the patient's head and place your feet on the outside corners of his shoulders. Then, as if you were riding a bicycle, push one shoulder downward with your foot, then the other. This relaxes the patient and helps a stiff neck.

Since you may often have pains in the neck, and there isn't always a Shiatsu practitioner available to relieve it, it is helpful to learn to give your own neck Shiatsu.

Self-Shiatsu Techniques

When you give Shiatsu to your neck, press softly at first and then more strongly. With your four fingers try rubbing, pushing, and pulling with a rhythmic motion on the back of your neck. Work for five minutes on one side, then five minutes on the other (Fig. 6–9). Then, with your thumb, press A Mon (Governing Vessel #15). Press hard and upward for five seconds, then release. Do this three times. You can find A Mon by locating the indentation in the center of the neck.

Intertwine your fingers and with your elbows forward, place your hands on the back of your neck. Massage the neck by squeezing your palms toward one another on the back of your neck (Fig. 6–10). Don't pull forward on the neck; just squeeze your palms. All these techniques loosen up tension and tightness.

FIG. 6–9
NECK
SELF-SHIATSU—RUBBING
THE NECK WITH
FOUR FINGERS

FIG. 6–10
NECK
SELF-SHIATSU—MASSAGING
THE NECK WITH
FINGERS INTERTWINED

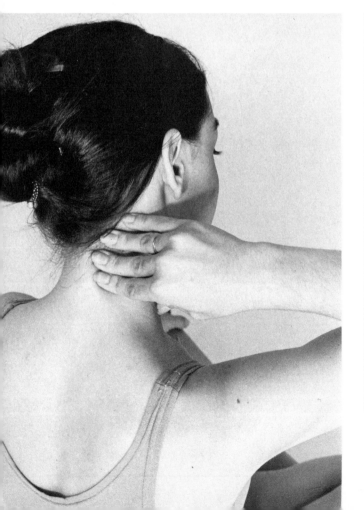

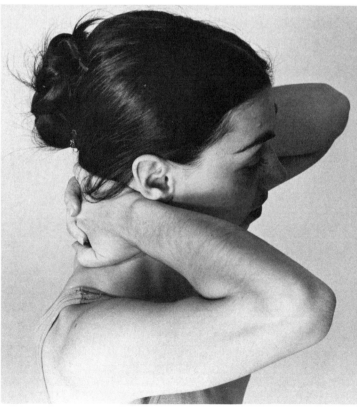

7. Leg and Foot Shiatsu

Have you ever noticed that a ballerina looks much younger than other people her age? Since I treat dancers regularly I am constantly amazed to see how they preserve and maintain a youthful appearance—until they stop dancing. The minute a dancer retires he usually begins to age almost immediately, and his health starts to deteriorate as well. This should tell you how important it is to keep ki-energy flowing through the feet and legs. The reason dancers stay young and vigorous is that their legs are constantly in action; when they stop dancing they age because they are no longer using their legs any more than the rest of us. Oriental doctors have long believed that deterioration begins in the legs.

The legs may seem mere appendages to the rest of the body, but, in fact, they are closely connected to the vital organs by the three Yin and three Yang meridians that run up and down the legs. The leg muscles come up to the Hara and the back muscles go down to the legs—so lower-back ache and stomach pain are often related to energy stagnation in the legs. There are also many important nerves in the legs, and nerve endings from organs and muscles in the entire body are located in the feet, which is why we can both diagnose and treat ailments in the body simply by massaging the feet.

Any doubts you may still have about the existence of the meridian lines should disappear when you recall the stories about people who lose a leg yet still feel pain in it when the weather is changing. We call this "phantom pain," and it is felt because the meridians in the other leg still exist and are connected to an invisible aura of energy in the absent limb. We can even treat "phantom pain" by pressing tsubos in the leg that remains.

In modern society few of us walk unless we have to, so energy stagnates easily in the feet and legs. Leg and foot Shiatsu is a must to compensate for our lack of exercise and for keeping not only the legs, but the rest of the body healthy.

How to Give Leg Shiatsu

First warm up the patient's legs by squeezing the muscles upward along the thighs, calves, and shinbones.

93

STRETCHING THE HIP AND THIGH

To ease general fatigue and tired legs have the patient lie on his side with the top leg bent. Put one hand on his hip and the other on his thigh and stretch in opposite directions (Fig. 7–1).

STEPPING ON THE BACKS OF THE THIGHS

Have the patient lie on his stomach. Bend each of his legs 90 degrees and step on the upper part of the back of his thighs (Fig. 7–2). You may also step on both thighs at the same time, keeping your balance by holding onto the patient's feet. Be sure not to step on the back of his knees. For energizing tired legs.

PRESSING TSUBOS IN THE LEGS

You can, of course, press tsubos on all the leg meridians (consult the chart in chapter 2 for exact locations) but there are several specific tsubos

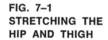

**FIG. 7–1
STRETCHING THE
HIP AND THIGH**

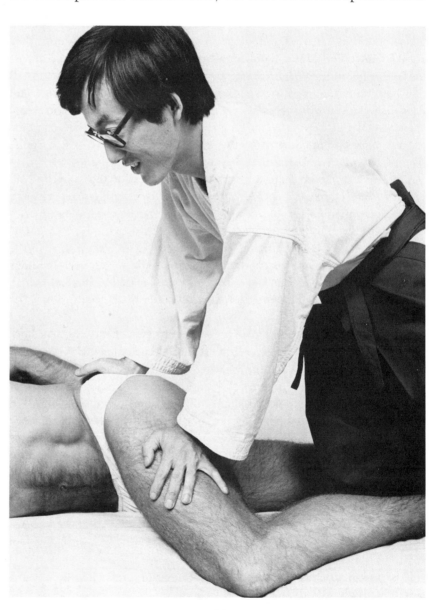

which are especially important to treat for tired legs and general health.

GALL BLADDER #31. The patient lies on his side with his top leg bent at the knee. Press Gall Bladder #31 (located on the side of each thigh at the tip of the middle finger when the patient stands with his arms at his sides) with one thumb on top of the other, gently, three times (Fig. 7–3, see p. 96). This helps poor circulation and tired legs. Remember to press the point on both thighs.

STOMACH #36. This is one of the most important tsubos in the human body; it is good for almost everything, including revitalizing ki-energy in the body. It is located just below the kneecap and off the shinbone on the outside of the leg. Press inward with one thumb (Fig. 7–4, see p. 96). If you want to ease the pressure you can vibrate the hand. If you need more pressure, ask the patient to bend one leg and then press using both thumbs, one on top of the other. You can and should press Stomach #36 in your own legs.

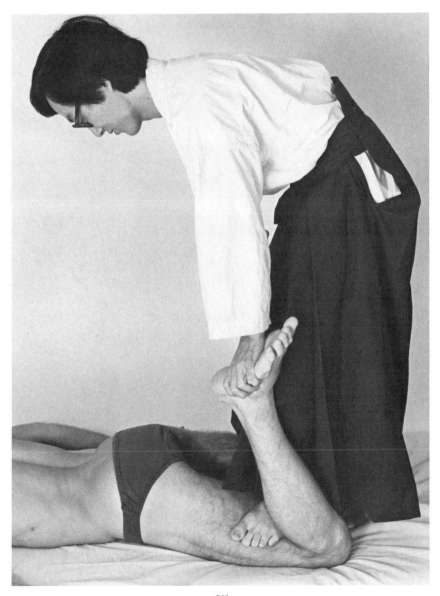

FIG. 7–2
STEPPING ON THE
BACKS OF THE
THIGHS

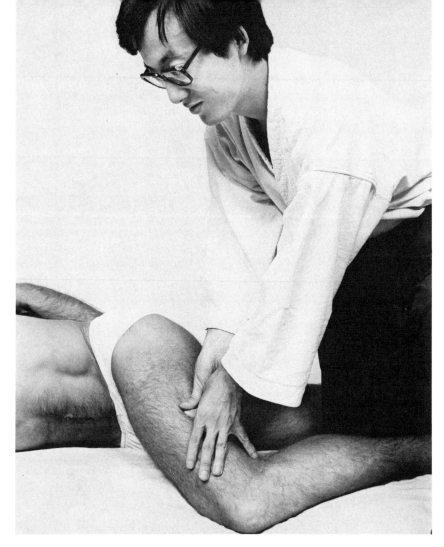

**FIG. 7–3
PRESSING
GALL BLADDER #31**

**FIG. 7–4
PRESSING
STOMACH #36**

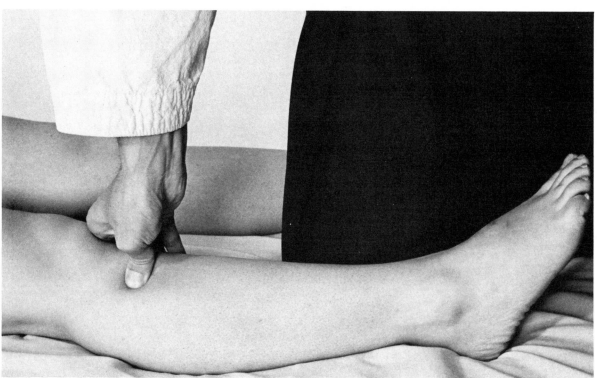

BLADDER MERIDIAN TSUBOS IN THE LEGS

Consult the chart in chapter 2 again to review the important Bladder Meridian tsubos in the legs. In Fig. 7–5 I am pressing the Bladder Meridian points in the back of the thigh, using one thumb on top of the other. This will help backache, sciatica, sexual, and digestion problems.

Knee Shiatsu

Americans are more prone to knee problems than Japanese because they are taller and heavier, and they get less exercise—all of which makes the knee fragile and liable to deteriorate. Keep your own knees in shape by stretching the leg and "moving" the kneecap with your fingers as much as possible. Then press inward on the area all around the kneecap, or the edge of the kneecap.

**FIG. 7–5
PRESSING BLADDER
MERIDIAN TSUBOS
IN THE LEGS**

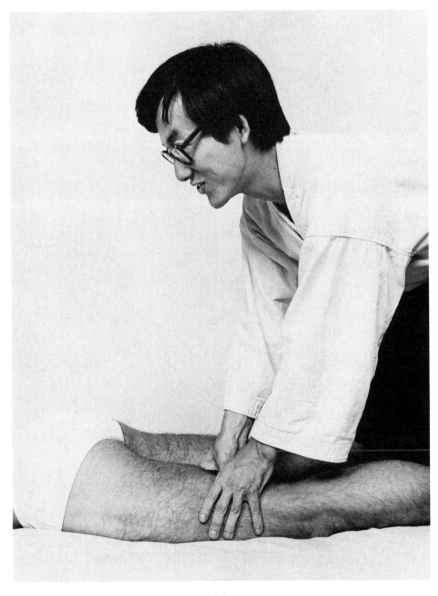

97

Hip Shiatsu

In general, massaging the hips relieves lower-back ache, sexual problems, and tired legs. First, relax the patient by vibrating, circulating, and pressing the muscles in the upper part of the buttocks, or sacrum area, using three or four fingers of both hands while the patient is on his stomach (Fig. 7–6).

SQUEEZING THE MUSCLES ON THE HIPS

Bend the patient's legs at the knees and support them in that position with your own legs. Then, using your palms, squeeze the muscles of the hips up and toward each other (Fig. 7–7). Do this three to five times.

**FIG. 7–6
MASSAGING THE HIPS
WITH FOUR FINGERS**

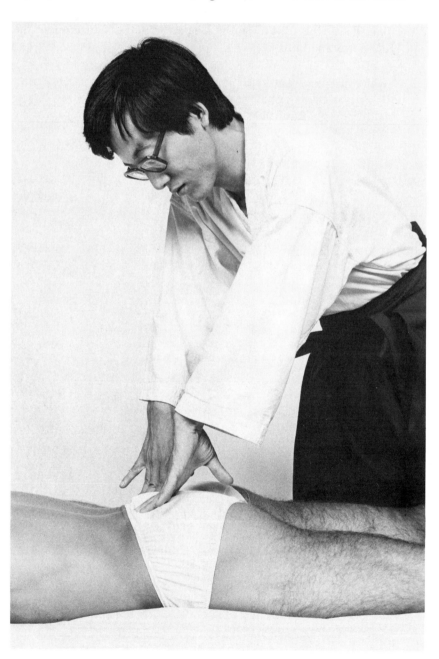

PRESSING TEN SHI AND GALL BLADDER #30

There are two important tsubos in the hips, Ten Shi and Gall Bladder #30. The patient can lie on his stomach while you kneel behind him and press the tsubos in toward the center of the body. It is too painful to press these sensitive points on both sides at the same time, so press one and then the other. For more pressure, lean hard into the tsubo by placing one leg between the patient's legs and keeping your arms stretched (Fig. 7–8, see p. 100). However, if the patient is big, heavy, or muscular, you can ask him to lie on his side, and then kneel beside him, putting all of your weight into the tsubo (Fig. 7–9, see p. 100).

The Ten Shi point is not on any of the meridian lines. It is located about three inches to the side of the patient's hipbone on the buttocks. Remem-

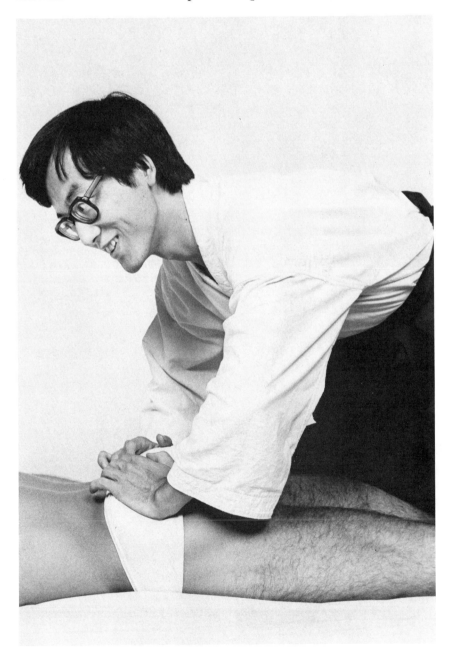

FIG. 7–7
SQUEEZING THE
MUSCLES
ON THE HIPS

99

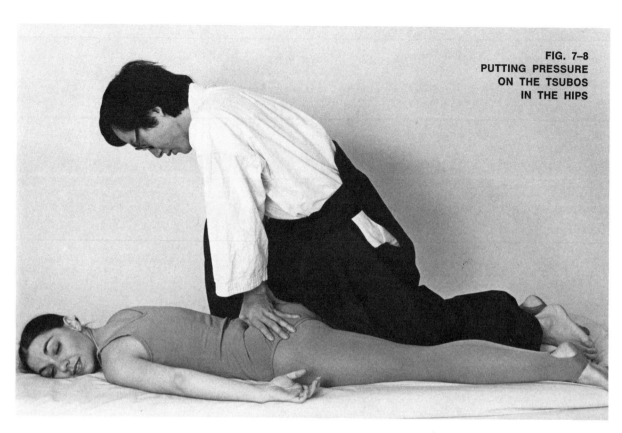

FIG. 7–8
PUTTING PRESSURE
ON THE TSUBOS
IN THE HIPS

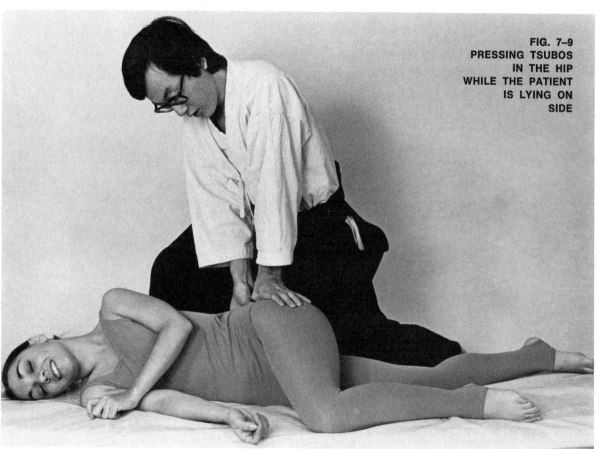

FIG. 7–9
PRESSING TSUBOS
IN THE HIP
WHILE THE PATIENT
IS LYING ON
SIDE

ber to press one tsubo at a time, in toward the sacrum, for 10–15 seconds, three times, for lower-back ache, sexual strength, and digestion. If you have trouble finding the point, place your fingers on the hipbone and stretch your thumb up toward the buttocks. If you bend the patient's knees with your other hand the point will be easier to find (Fig. 7–10).

Gall Bladder #30 (not pictured in the preceding illustrations) is lower on the buttocks than Ten Shi and closer to the center of the body. Press the same way you pressed Ten Shi, bending the patient's legs to help you find the point, for lower-back ache, numbness in the legs, and sciatica. (See chapter 2 for exact location.)

Reflexology or Foot Shiatsu

The nerves from all the important organs have extremely sensitive endings in the feet. Even nerves from the brain go straight to the feet, which

FIG. 7–10
FINDING TEN SHI

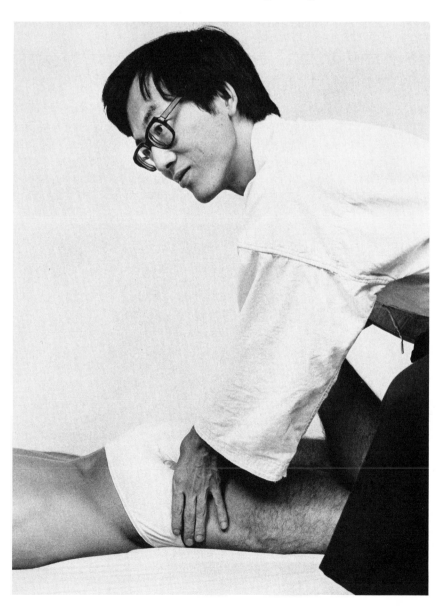

is why we can treat mental disorders by massaging them. If you doubt this fact, the simplest way to prove it to yourself is to find someone with poor vision and press hard on the inside of his big toe, the part of the foot where the eyes have their nerve endings. He will probably scream with pain; a person with good vision will feel almost no pain at all.

The best way to approach foot Shiatsu is to imagine the sole of the foot as a miniature model of the human body. The toes represent the head, eyes, ears, and nose; the ball of the foot represents the organs of the solar plexus (liver, gall bladder, pancreas, and stomach); the area beneath the arch, the kidney, transverse colon, and small intestine; and the part of the sole just under the heel, the sexual organs. Theoretically, you can diagnose ailments and treat them by massaging the part of the foot that corresponds to the malfunctioning organ. If exceptional pain and stiffness occur anywhere in the foot, the organ represented by that area is having trouble. My own view, however, is that it is more important to massage the feet for general health and revitalization of energy than for specific, localized problems. If you thoroughly massage both feet, you'll automatically treat any ailment the patient may have, whether you try or not.

You should massage hard each foot separately with a hooked thumb or knuckle of the middle finger, digging into the foot for about fifteen minutes. In a proper foot massage the patient *should* feel pain, even a lot of pain, as if sharp points are entering his foot. Concentrate on the sole and the areas between the toes; then pinch the Achilles tendon strongly to stimulate sex glands, kidneys, and bladder, and dig four fingers deeply into the heel bone on the sole to activate sex glands and relieve backache and stiff knees. Insomnia and nervous tension can be relieved by massaging

FG. 7–11
SOLE TO SOLE

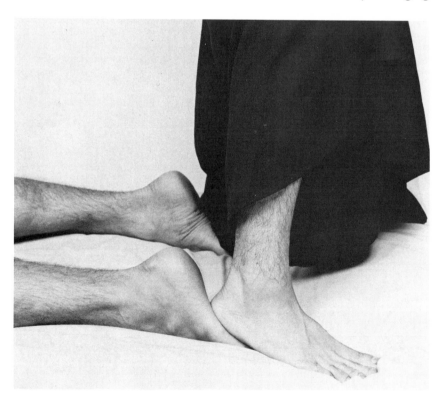

102

the middle of the sole, under the arch. You can, of course, massage your own feet the same way—an easy way to keep your body in top condition.

SOLE TO SOLE

A pleasant way to stimulate the feet, relax nervous tension, and communicate with a friend is to lie on your stomach, open your legs, and ask a friend to step on the soles of your feet with his (Fig. 7–11). He should make sure not to step on your heel. If there is an arc between the knee and the ankle, a pillow should be placed under the shinbone. This simple exercise is very effective and a highly personal means of communication, strange though it may seem. As one of my students remarked, "You understand more about the person you're stepping on than he could tell you about himself." You can vary this exercise by kneeling on the soles of your friend's feet and massaging his thighs and calves at the same time. This promotes a feeling of comfort and well-being (Fig. 7–12).

**FIG. 7–12
KNEELING
ON THE SOLES
AND MASSAGING
THE THIGHS**

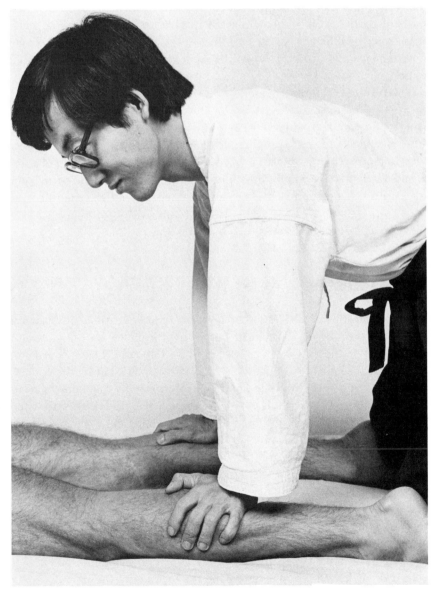

8. Arm and Chest Shiatsu

The arms, like the legs, may seem to be mere "attachments" to the vital parts of the body. But it is important to give arm Shiatsu for the same reasons we give Shiatsu to the legs. In fact, many thousands of years ago, before man stood upright, the arms were legs because man walked on all fours.

Three Yang and three Yin meridians connect the arms to the organs and muscles in the torso. On the inside of the arms run the Heart, Lung, and Heart Constrictor meridians (Yin), and on the outside run the Large Intestine, Small Intestine, and Triple Heater meridians (Yang). The best way to approach arm Shiatsu is to review these meridian lines in chapter 2 and then practice finding and pressing the important tsubos in your own arms or your patient's. You can also massage all the meridians at once by pressing both sides of the patient's arms with your palms, moving them up and down the arm.

Large Intestine #4 and #10

Large Intestine #10 is another important point to press for general health and well-being. To find it, put your little finger on the crease of your elbow on the outside. This is Large Intestine #11. Leave your hand where it is. Beneath your middle finger, three inches down the arm, is Large Intestine #10. Find the point and catch it with your thumb. Hold your own (or the patient's) arm lightly and move it back and forth while you are pressing (Fig. 8–1). Press for 10–15 seconds, three times.

In Fig. 8–2 the model is pressing Large Intestine #4 in her own hand, an important point for treating headaches, rashes, toothaches, and facial tension. She has found the point by putting her thumb in the space between the thumb and forefinger of the other hand and bending it at the first joint. The tip of her thumb then touches the fleshy mound between these two fingers, or Large Intestine #4. Press this point toward the index finger on yourself or the patient for 10–15 seconds, three times. If you are working on a patient, be sure to use his fingers to find these points, not your own, as his proportions determine the location of the point.

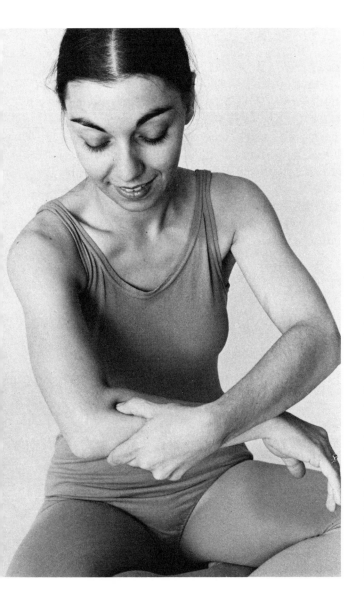 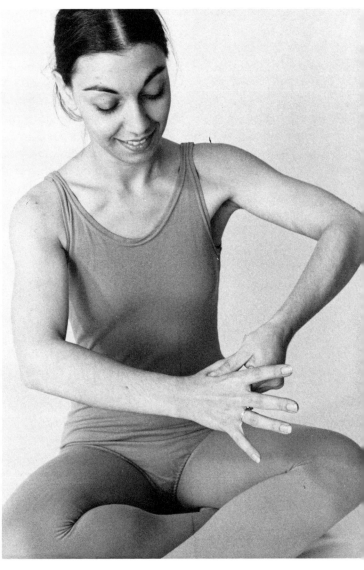

Finger Shiatsu

**FIG. 8–1
PRESSING LARGE
INTESTINE #10**

**FIG. 8–2
PRESSING LARGE
INTESTINE #4**

In Japan merchants teach their apprentices to rub their fingers and palms when customers irritate them; this relieves the tension caused by difficult sales transactions. You can practice this kind of self-Shiatsu on your own fingers. To relieve tension in the hands and bring about a feeling of relaxation and well-being, press the knuckle of one finger of your right hand with the thumb and index finger of your left. Now pull with a shaking movement, gradually sliding your thumb and index finger away from the knuckle. Give the tip of the finger a final pinch and go on to the next finger. Then change hands. You can do the same exercise by bending the index and middle fingers and grasping the finger to be massaged between them. Apply pressure the same way as in the first exercise. You can give the same treatment to your patient. Since so many meridian lines end in the fingertips, the process of giving Shiatsu will stimulate them and make your whole body stronger.

Chest Shiatsu

The respiratory and circulatory functions take place in the chest, controlled by two vital organs—the heart and the lungs. Chest Shiatsu stimulates the heart and the lungs, relieves muscle pain in the chest and the shoulders, improves lactation in nursing mothers and makes healthy milk for their babies. In Japan we have special masseuses who work only on the chest areas of nursing mothers.

In America breast cancer is a great enemy of women; fortunately, it can almost always be arrested if it is detected early. Chest Shiatsu keeps your patient aware of changes in the chest area; if you feel abnormal stiffness or small lumps, like kidney beans, in the chest while you are being massaged (or massaging), go to a physician immediately.

TRACING THE RIB CAGE

The chest area is soft and fragile, so you must be careful to press gently. Have the patient lie on his back and relax. Open your four fingers and place them between the ribs on the rib cage. Then draw the flesh from

FIG. 8–3
TRACING THE RIB CAGE

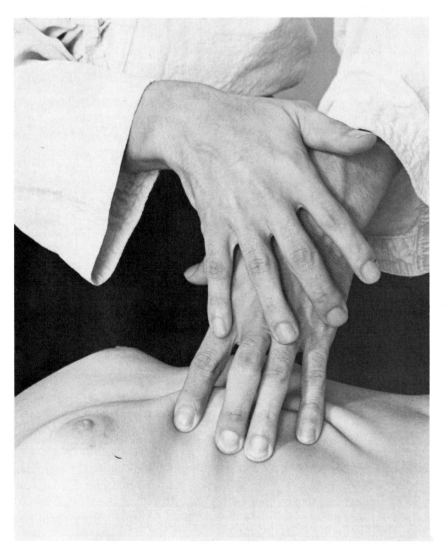

the center of the rib cage out to the sides. Press down and pull out (Fig. 8-3). In the illustration I appear to be moving the flesh toward the rib cage; this is an optical illusion, as I am actually moving my fingers out toward the sides of the torso. You can do this to your own rib cage, as well as to your patient's.

PRESSING THE CENTER BONE

Place one thumb on top of the other and resting your palms across the patient's breast, press very gently on the center bone of the chest when he is exhaling. Press three to five times, for 5–7 seconds each time. For pain in the chest, palpitations, and lactation (Fig. 8-4).

PRESSING ALONG THE COLLARBONE

For a patient suffering from chest pains due to cold or flu, or frozen shoulder, put one thumb on top of the other and trace the area just beneath the collarbone, pressing in gently. These points are sensitive, but they are not tsubos. Press each area for 5–7 seconds, three times (Fig. 8-5).

**FIG. 8–4
PRESSING THE
CENTER BONE**

**FIG. 8–5
PRESSING ALONG
THE COLLAR BONE**

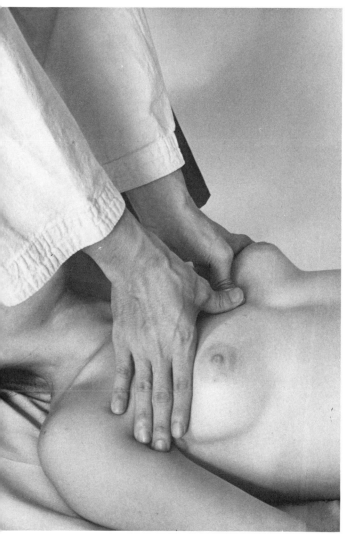

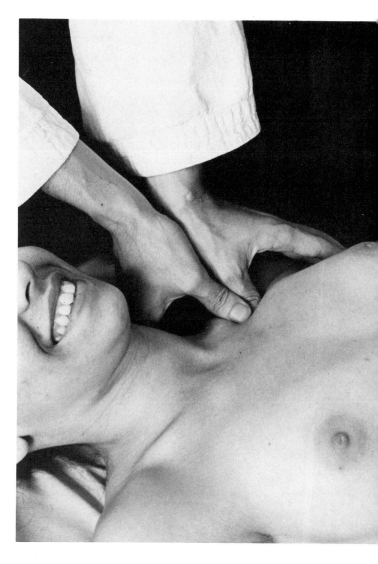

107

9. Face and Ear Shiatsu

There is an English expression, "Beauty is only skin deep." In my opinion, however, a truly beautiful face goes far deeper than the surface—it is the reflection of good physical, emotional, and mental health, not makeup, a suntan, or the right kind of moisturizing cream, as so many magazine advertisements would ask us to believe. Pimples, rashes, eczema, and poor skin tone represent an unhealthy condition somewhere in the body which can be corrected by diet, exercise, and Shiatsu. We can also create and sculpture our faces according to the lives we live, the emotions we experience, the work we do, and how we educate ourselves. Especially after forty, when the natural beauty of youth begins to fade, we must take responsibility for our faces. If we are trusted by others, our faces look trustworthy; if we are frustrated, we look frustrated, and no eyeshadow in the world will make us appear beautiful. The meaning of "inner beauty" is never more evident to me than when I see one of my women patients growing more healthy or falling sincerely in love—her face develops a good, healthy, shining color and that alone makes her beautiful to me.

Shiatsu treatments on the entire body will improve facial beauty by helping to stimulate the functions of the major organs and eliminate tension which causes bad skin, facial lines, and a nervous, dissatisfied expression. We also have Shiatsu techniques especially for the face which improve not only facial beauty, but the condition of the body as a whole.

Skin Diagnosis

In the Orient we have established methods of diagnosing health and character by examining the color, structure, and lines of the face. The color tone of facial skin, we believe, is strongly affected by the condition of the liver, heart, spleen, lungs, kidneys, and to a lesser degree by their associated organs, the gall bladder, small intestine, stomach, large intestine, and bladder. People with red-toned faces—especially in the center of the nose—may suffer heart trouble. A yellowish face indicates a spleen or pancreas problem. A lung problem is revealed by a white color on the face. Kidney trouble is indicated by a dark, blackish color and sometimes by freckles. A greenish skin tone and yellowish eyes can mean liver problems. When people with liver trouble drink alcohol, their faces become pale or blue instead of flushed. Before leaping to conclusions give other diagnostic tests for the organs. Don't confuse a natural olive, rosy, or dark skin tone with an unnatural hue; compare what you consider an abnormal skin tone to the patient's usual color.

The upper, middle, and lower parts of the face correspond to the upper, middle, and lower parts of the torso. If the skin of each part is bright, smooth, and flexible, the corresponding part of the body is healthy. Poor color or texture, blemishes, dark marks, or wrinkles in a young person, or any unusual condition, such as a severely twisted jaw, indicate difficulties in the corresponding part of the body.

Blemishes

Blemishes trouble a great many people in Westernized or affluent countries. In an underdeveloped country like India, where little meat and sugar are consumed, one almost never sees a case of acne. In the East we believe that pimples and blemishes are caused by hormonal imbalance during adolescence, menstrual irregularity in women, or toxins in the body caused by improper diet, digestive malfunctions, and especially by constipation, one of the skin's worst enemies. Often, the cure is to stop using makeup, change the diet from animal protein to vegetables, seaweed, and grains, and cut off all sugar. Give yourself Ampuku therapy (chapter 5) to stimulate digestion and regular bowel movements.

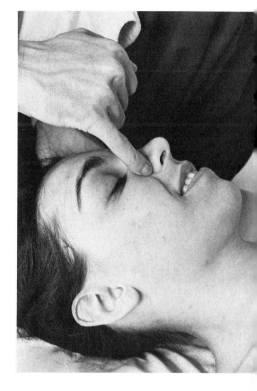

FIG. 9–1
PRESSING LARGE INTESTINE #20

FIG. 9–2
PRESSING STOMACH #3

Face Shiatsu

Review your study of the meridian lines in the face in chapter 2 to locate the important tsubos. Many of the tsubos in the face are small and hard to reach, in grooves near the eyes or nose that are not easily accessible. In Fig. 9–1 I am demonstrating how to use the little finger when pressing Large Intestine #20 on the side of the nose. Press for 5–7 seconds, three times, for nasal stagnation and sinus congestion, great hindrances to facial beauty.

STOMACH #3

Kyo Sho, another excellent point for clearing sinuses and nasal stagnation, is located near the side of the nose and directly below the pupils when they are looking straight ahead. Press hard and inward toward the eye with your thumb or index finger. Be careful not to slip and jab the eye (Fig. 9–2).

TAI YO

Tai Yo, one finger's width away from the end of the eyebrow, between the eyebrow and the outer edge of the eye, relieves headache and tired

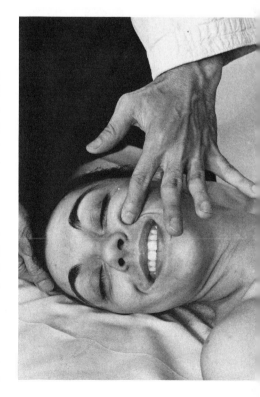

eyes when pressed hard and inward for 7–10 seconds, three times (Fig. 9–3).

GOVERNING VESSEL MERIDIAN

The Governing Vessel Meridian is located in the center of the forehead, just above the eyebrows and In Do. With one thumb on top of the other press hard and inward for 5–7 seconds, three to five times, for headache and nervous tension. Pressing the Governing Vessel point can stimulate new hair growth, too (Fig. 9–4).

Other Important Tsubos for the Face

Stomach #9, located one and a half inches from the middle of the larynx, where a small pulse is felt, can relieve hypertension and stimulate the thyroid gland and production of hormones (which beautify the skin). Press softly and inward with one thumb for 10–15 seconds, three times.

Bladder #23 and #52 (located in the back; see chapter 2, Bladder Meridian tsubos) are important points for promoting kidney functions and giving life energy to the body, which is reflected in the color and skin tone of the face. A healthy kidney is also necessary for good hearing.

IN DO

The point which we call In Do, located on the forehead between the eyebrows, is the same point Indian people call the "third eye." They believe this is the place where your soul appears, which is why Indian women adorn it with a colored dot. The In Do, according to Oriental theory, is the mirror of the body's health. If you have a bright, smooth, and flexible In Do, you are in basically good condition; even if you are sick or critically wounded, a healthy In Do indicates you will survive. The same point appears, we believe, like a dot, visible on the forehead, when you are about to die. Press the In Do hard and inward with two thumbs for 7–10 seconds, three times, to relieve headache and nasal obstruction (see the chart in chapter 2 for exact location).

Tracing Lines in the Face

One of the best ways to remove wrinkles and ease facial tension is to place your fingers on different areas of your face and move the skin in an outward or upward direction, tracing imaginary "lines" in the face with your fingers (see Figs. 9–5 and 9–6). Here are several tracing exercises you can give yourself or your patient:

1. Place four fingers on the outside of the nose near the base and move them outward toward the ears and jawbone along the chinbone.

2. Trace lines from the inside corners of the eyes to the upper part of the ears.

3. Trace lines from the tops of the eyebrows to the hairline, moving your fingers upward on the forehead.

4. Trace lines from the center of the jaw to the tips of the ears.

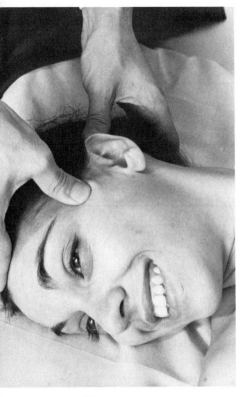

**FIG. 9–3
PRESSING TAI YO**

**FIG. 9–4
PRESSING GOVERNING
VESSEL MERIDIAN**

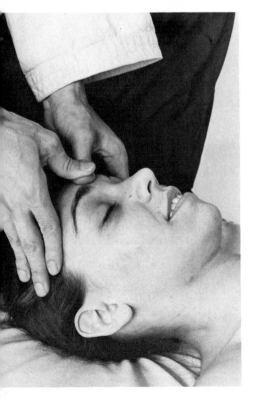

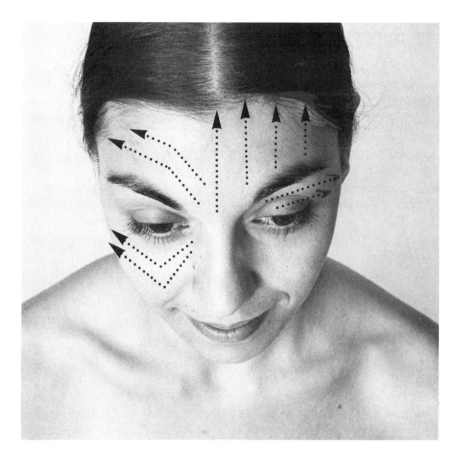

FIG. 9–5
TRACING LINES
IN THE FACE

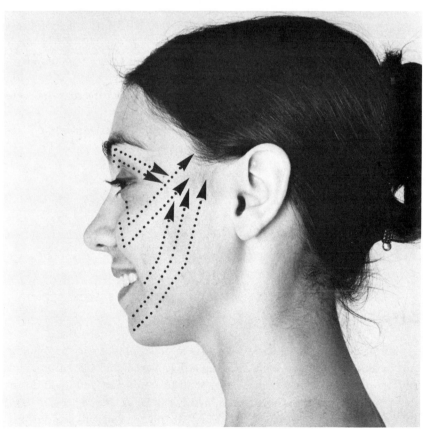

FIG. 9–6
TRACING LINES
IN THE FACE

111

Self-Shiatsu for the Face

There are several Shiatsu techniques you can use on your face which stimulate many meridians at once and relax tension. Rub your hands vigorously to warm them and rub the palms briskly on the cheeks, up and down. This massages the Stomach Meridian and the Small Intestine Meridian at the same time. Then rub the cheekbones and the sides of the nose energetically with your fingers to stimulate the Stomach Meridian, which begins just below the eye, and the Bladder Meridian, which begins on each side of the nose. The fists can be used like small hammers to beat the scalp lightly, invigorating the Bladder, Gall Bladder, and Triple Heater meridians (just above the ears). To prevent a double chin from forming, hook the thumbs and dig them under the jawbone, massaging deeply. If you feel pain or if hard flesh is in evidence, it is a sign you are eating too much. Massage regularly to make the flesh soft.

Eye Shiatsu

DIAGNOSIS

In Oriental medicine we say that the eye is the mirror of the liver. If your eyes are extremely sensitive to light, if they tear abnormally, get tired easily, discharge, or have a yellow color, your liver may be malfunctioning. A bluish color below the eyes can indicate weak kidneys, caused by overindulgence in sex, lack of sleep, or overwork.

Abnormally enlarged pupils also indicate bad health. In a healthy person's eye the pupil is surrounded by white only on top and on the sides. If there is a white area beneath the pupil we say the eye is *Sanpaku*—the sign of a very unhealthy person or a corpse.

Here is a series of massages to relax tired eyes and decrease nervous tension:

1. Rub your hands together hard and rapidly to make them warm. Place them on your own, or your patient's eyes, very gently (Fig. 9–7).

2. Put four fingers on the closed eyes and make small, gentle, circular movements (Fig. 9–8).

3. Place three fingers on the upper lid of the eye. Press gently upward (Fig. 9–9).

4. Finally, put your thumbs on the closed eyes, applying very gentle pressure (Fig. 9–10).

Ear Shiatsu

The ear is today considered by acupuncturists one of the most important parts of the human body. We have discovered that the ear contains tiny Acupuncture points which correspond to every part and organ in the body; many kinds of diseases and ailments can be diagnosed and treated by inserting needles in them. If you look at the ear you will see that it is

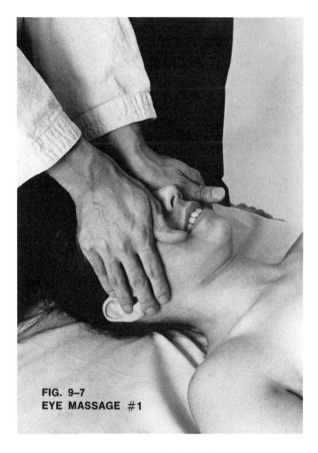

FIG. 9–7
EYE MASSAGE #1

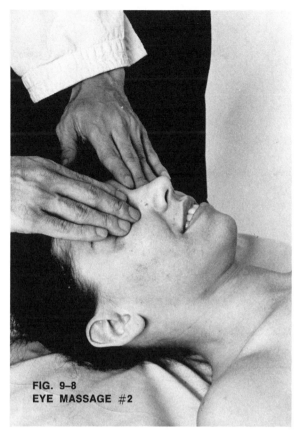

FIG. 9–8
EYE MASSAGE #2

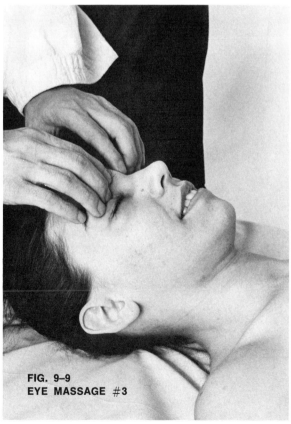

FIG. 9–9
EYE MASSAGE #3

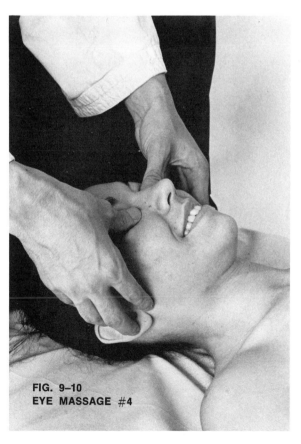

FIG. 9–10
EYE MASSAGE #4

113

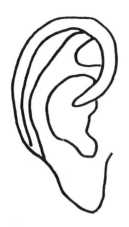

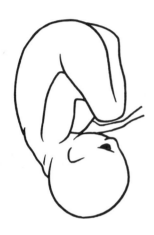

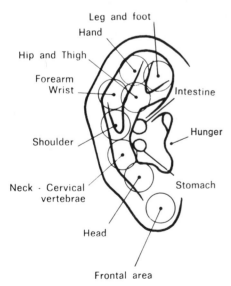

Leg and foot
Hand
Hip and Thigh
Forearm
Wrist
Intestine
Shoulder
Hunger
Neck - Cervical
vertebrae
Stomach
Head
Frontal area

**FIG. 9–11
DIAGRAMS OF
ACUPUNCTURE POINTS
IN THE EAR**

shaped exactly like a human embryo, which may suggest the reason why it is a microcosm of the whole body.

In auricular therapy needles are inserted into the ear points; in Shiatsu we press them with toothpicks or another slender instrument to apply stimulation to the tiny tsubos. This method of treatment may be older than we think. Pirates, for example, have always worn bones or earrings in the ears in exactly the place where the eye acu-point is located. This point can be stimulated and vision improved by making a hole where it is located. (This no doubt helped the pirates to see long distances, so necessary for their careers.) Recently Acupuncture doctors have discovered that damaging habits such as smoking and overeating can be halted when a kind of staple is placed in a certain point in the ear and left there. Seventy percent of the overweight patients treated by one acupuncturist with this staple reported decreased appetite and weight loss. When a patient wearing the staple feels a hunger urge, he merely wiggles it and this keeps his impetus under control. Acupuncturists are experimenting with this method to cure drug addiction, too.

HOW TO GIVE AURICULAR THERAPY

First examine the diagram of Acupuncture points on the auricle. (Fig. 9–11), then press lightly around the ear with a pointed object like a toothpick. If there is abnormal pain or extreme sensitivity at any point in the ear there may be a problem in the corresponding area of the body; for example if there is pain in the shoulder point, the patient may have shoulder pain. To treat the ailment continue pressing the point with a pecking motion with the toothpick until pain disappears or decreases in the point. You can, of course, augment the effectiveness of your treatment by applying other Shiatsu techniques which affect the same area of the body. You must of course, be very careful not to pierce or in any way injure the ear.

HOW TO LOSE WEIGHT WITH AURICULAR THERAPY

Although acupuncturists inject a staple in the stomach and hunger points to help patients lose weight, we can also decrease hunger yearnings with ear Shiatsu. Whenever you feel hungry press these points with a toothpick.

EAR DIAGNOSIS

Orientals believe that the bigger the ear, the longer life, better health and fortune you will have. The Buddha was said to have very large ears with long earlobes. Well-balanced, thick, round ears are a sign of good health. Japanese children often have their ears pulled, not as punishment, but to help them achieve a rich, healthy, and long life. Clean and shining ears are also supposed to bring good fortune.

Kidney trouble is reflected in the ears. Poor hearing, ear pain, and ringing in the ears are often caused by kidney problems. A bluish or dark-colored ear is also a signal that the kidney is malfunctioning. If you have these symptoms you should be checked by a specialist. Even if there is an external or mechanical reason for the problem, you should still check your kidneys and other organs.

PRESSING TRIPLE HEATER TSUBOS
WITH THUMB AND LITTLE FINGER

For ear problems of any kind you can press Triple Heater #21, on the side of the ear, with your thumb for 5–7 seconds, three to five times (Fig. 9–12), or Triple Heater #17, in the small groove just below the earlobe, with your little finger (Fig. 9–13).

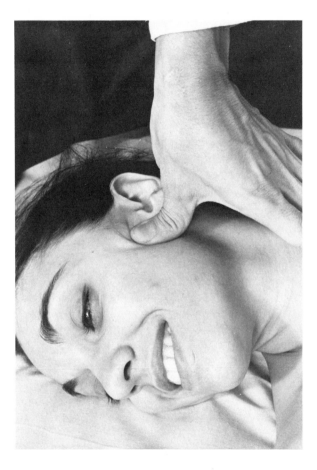

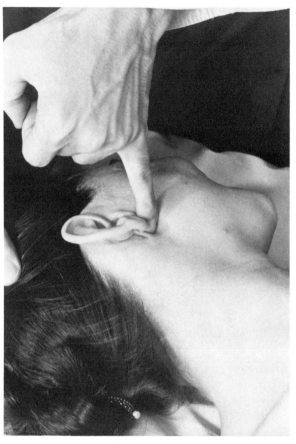

FIG. 9–12
PRESSING TRIPLE
HEATER #21

FIG. 9–13
PRESSING TRIPLE
HEATER #17

10. Shiatsu Exercise

We all know the importance of exercise in our lives. Without exercise our bodies atrophy and decay; our joints and muscles become stiff and painful; the heart grows sluggish; and since the heart pumps the blood, the circulation grows sluggish too. And of course one of the most unpleasant symptoms of lack of exercise—the one we are usually forced to recognize first—is added fat. As the body atrophies the slightest effort to exert ourselves creates pain and fatigue in the muscles and joints. As the circulation and nervous systems decline the organs they support also suffer and we become prone to nervous disorders and tension. We can't sleep at night; we are cranky and irritable. We look, feel, and act older than we are.

In the West we try to stop the symptoms of atrophy with pills—pills to relieve insomnia, pills to relieve a tension headache, pills to increase the appetite, pills to decrease the appetite. From the Oriental point of view this is like trying to produce water in a dried-up reservoir by changing the washer in the faucet. Completely futile! We must fill the reservoir again with the ki-energy that Shiatsu, proper diet, and exercise help us to obtain.

Unfortunately, the many mechanical conveniences and innumerable desk jobs of contemporary life eliminate our greatest source of natural exercise—physical work. Cars make it unnecessary for us to walk—a vital kind of exercise—and there are too many forms of entertainment that offer us enjoyment without our moving our bodies at all. To compensate for all the ways society has made it possible for us to relax, we must design special kinds of work, or exercises, for our bodies to keep them young, healthy, and strong.

What, you may ask, is a chapter on exercise doing in a book about Shiatsu? Exercise, like Shiatsu, prevents ki-energy from stagnating in the body and gives you a means to keep energy flowing through the meridian lines via your own efforts. We also rely on exercise—stretching, rotating, and moving our muscles and limbs—to prevent the stagnation of ki-energy in the joints, where many important tsubos exist that are impossible to press with the fingers.

The exercises I recommend in this chapter have the same general benefits as Shiatsu treatments. Unlike typical Western exercises, which are designed to make one's body hard and muscular, these exercises make the body soft and flexible and facilitate the flow of ki-energy. The exercises I suggest implement the effectiveness of the Shiatsu treatment. One series you can do by yourself without any help. The other, especially beneficial for the back, must be done with the help of another person. Both kinds of exercise are easy, safe, and completely effective. You can do them before, after, or between Shiatsu treatments.

Exercises for Two

Most people hate to do exercises alone. Doing any kind of exercise with a friend to keep you company makes the time go faster and the pain less intense. Imagine, then, the added pleasure of having your friend help you move your body. When two people do exercises together the benefits for both are greater and the feeling of oneness between them is increased.

When you exercise alone your goal may be to relax and stretch, but ironically, your own exertions make you tense, and tension limits your ability to stretch. For this reason, someone else can stretch you more than you can stretch yourself, and relax you by taking control over your muscles.

The following simple exercises affect mainly the back, which must be stretched and flexible to stay healthy.

FIRST EXERCISE

Kneel beside your partner, who is lying on his back. Grasping the back of one ankle with your fingers, stretch his leg up and back toward his head as far as it will go (Fig. 10–1). Then do the same with the other

FIG. 10–1
EXERCISES FOR TWO:
FIRST EXERCISE

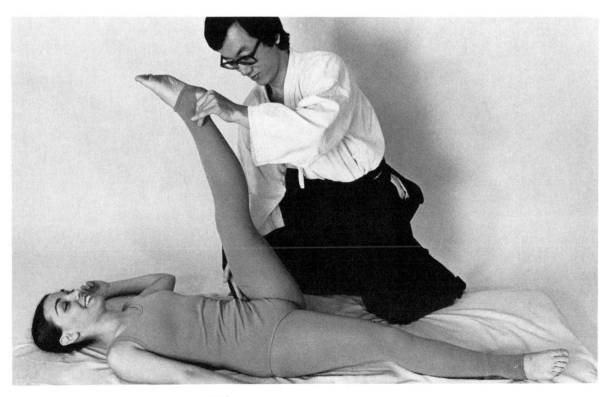

117

leg. This loosens the socket of the leg and also stretches the spinal muscle in the back.

SECOND EXERCISE

This is basically the same as the first exercise, except this time you grasp both of your partner's heels and stretch both legs back toward the head at the same time (Fig. 10–2).

THIRD EXERCISE

Hold your partner's toes in your left hand and with your right hand bend his knee and press it toward his head. Then rotate the knee clockwise and the toes counterclockwise simultaneously. Then reverse and rotate the knee counterclockwise and the toes clockwise (Fig. 10–3). Then do the same to his other leg.

FOURTH EXERCISE

Your partner sits on his heels as in the illustration and interlocks his fingers behind his head. You kneel behind him and place your knee in his back. Place your hands gently behind his ears without pressing. When he exhales pull his elbow back with your arms and at the same time push his head forward with your hands. Your knee will press into his back, stretching it (Fig. 10–4). Do this five times.

FIG. 10–2
EXERCISES FOR TWO:
SECOND EXERCISE

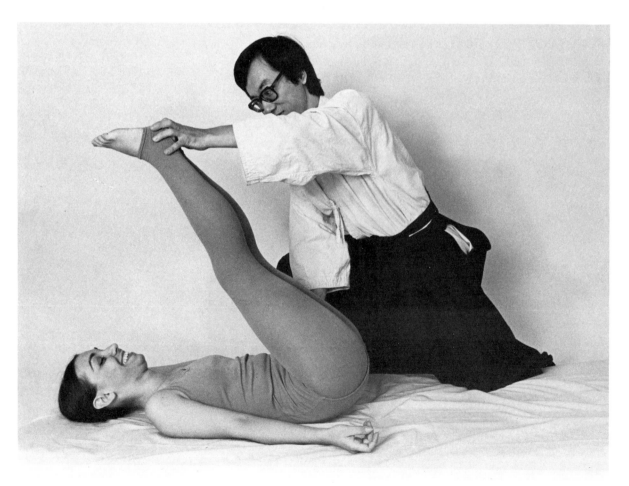

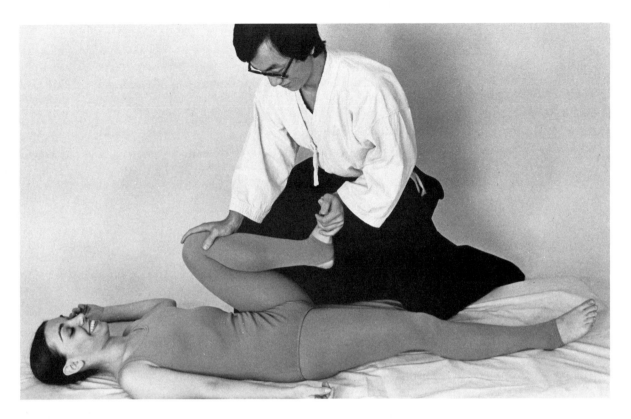

FIG. 10–3
EXERCISES FOR TWO:
THIRD EXERCISE

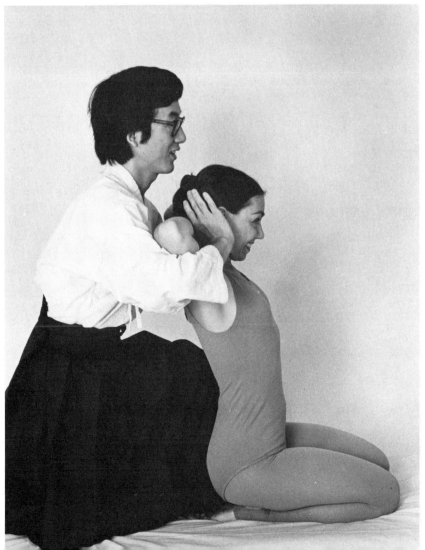

FIG. 10–4
EXERCISES FOR TWO:
FOURTH EXERCISE

FIFTH EXERCISE

Again, put your knee in your partner's back. This time his arms are stretched and your hands are placed on the back of his neck. When he exhales, pull his arms back with your arms as you gently push his neck forward with your hands (Fig. 10–5). Five times.

SIXTH EXERCISE

Again your partner sits on his heels with a straight back, interlocking his hands behind his head. You stand behind him with your knee in his back. When he exhales, pull his elbows back gently (Fig. 10–6). Make sure he's relaxed. Five times.

SEVENTH EXERCISE

This exercise is similar to the sixth, but gives your partner a more extreme stretch. He interlocks his fingers and you cup his hands in yours, as shown in the illustration. When he exhales, pull back his arms, which are straight, keeping your knee in his back as before (Fig. 10–7). Five times.

EIGHTH EXERCISE

Stand behind your partner, who is seated as before, and put your knee in his back. Grasp each of his hands in yours and when he exhales pull his straight arms back, opening the chest muscles and stretching the back and arms (Fig. 10–8). Do this five times.

NINTH EXERCISE

There are two ways to do this exercise. The first is to place your hand flat on top of your partner's head and then rotate it gently, first one way and then the other. This loosens the muscles in the neck. For a more extreme stretch, place your partner's head in the crook of your elbow and using your upper arm and forearm rotate it slowly and gently all the way around (Fig. 10–9; see p. 122 for Figs. 10–9 through 10–12). Don't stretch or crack his neck and spine. Tell him to relax and let you do the work. Two or three minutes.

TENTH EXERCISE

Stand back to back with your partner. Prepare for this exercise by linking arms at the elbow with your partner and separating your legs slightly (Fig. 10–10). Bend your knees (Fig. 10–11) and, bending forward and rounding your back, lift your partner up on your back (Fig. 10–12). Both of you should be relaxed; you should feel his weight in your legs and not in your back. You are stretching his back and stomach muscles; at the same time you are stretching your own back muscles and the muscles on the backs of the thighs.

Makko-Ho Exercises—For One Person

These four simple sitting exercises from Japan, called Makko-Ho, take just five minutes to do. They stretch the muscles and joints of your legs,

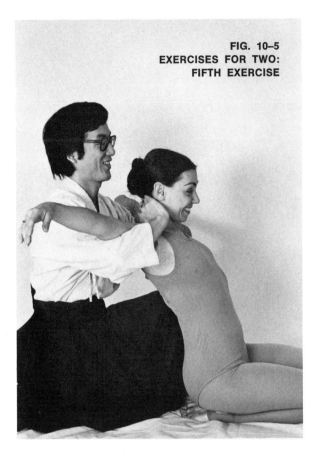

FIG. 10–5
EXERCISES FOR TWO:
FIFTH EXERCISE

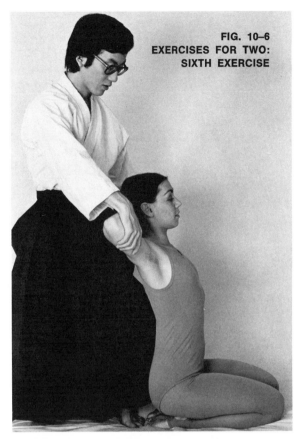

FIG. 10–6
EXERCISES FOR TWO:
SIXTH EXERCISE

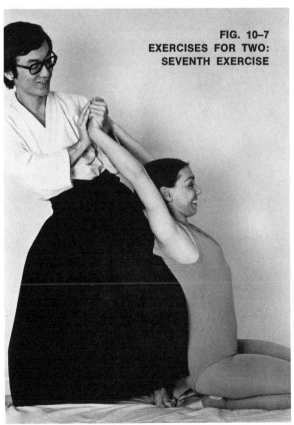

FIG. 10–7
EXERCISES FOR TWO:
SEVENTH EXERCISE

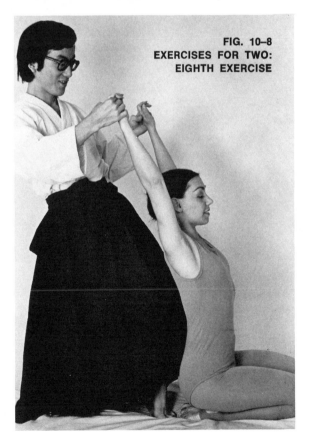

FIG. 10–8
EXERCISES FOR TWO:
EIGHTH EXERCISE

**FIG. 10–9
EXERCISES FOR TWO:
NINTH EXERCISE**

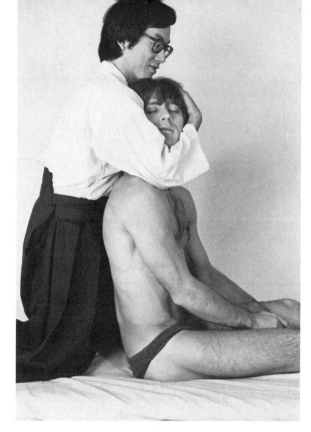

**FIGS. 10–10, 10–11
EXERCISES FOR TWO:
TENTH EXERCISE**

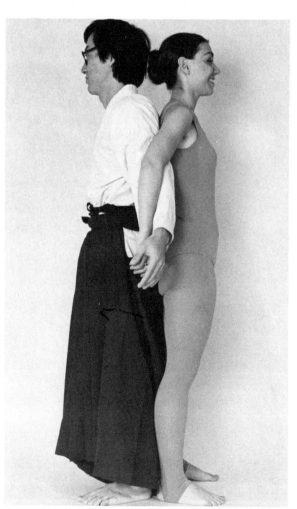

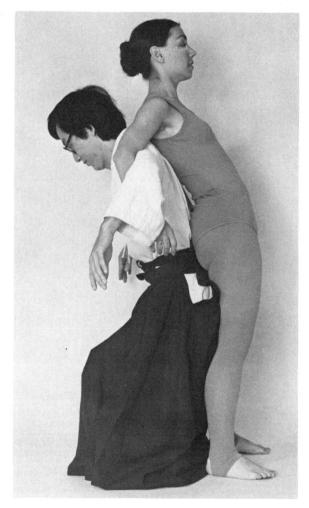

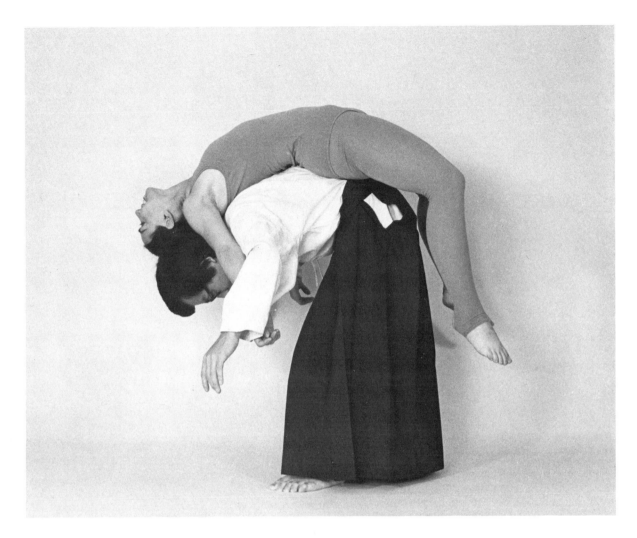

FIG. 10–12
EXERCISES FOR TWO:
TENTH EXERCISE

hips, and lower back. Makko-Ho exercises are especially valuable for the extremely stiff bodies of people who have not exercised for a long time. The aim of Makko-Ho is to return the body to the flexible state of a healthy child. (Small children, in fact, can do these exercises with no trouble at all, probably because they spend a great deal of time on the floor.)

You should do Makko-Ho on the floor once in the morning before breakfast and once again in the evening. If you have insomnia these exercises will help you sleep. If you do them after having too much to drink, they will ease your hangover. In the morning Makko-Ho is more painful, but it helps to wake you up and start your circulation going again. Be sure not to exaggerate the postures at first. Eventually you will be able to do them correctly without overstretching yourself.

EXERCISE ONE

Put the soles of your feet together and touch your knees to the floor. Now bend forward, extending the arms, until your head comes as close to the floor as possible (Figs. 10–13 and 10–14, see p. 124). This exercise stretches the spinal process (the jutting bones of the vertebrae) and opens the sockets of the legs. Do it ten or twenty times (but not if you're preg-

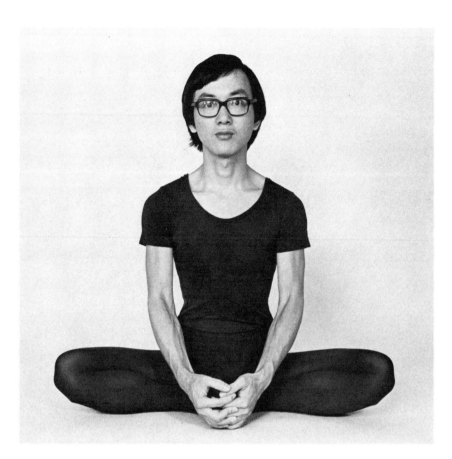

**FIGS. 10–13 AND 10–14
MAKKO-HO—
EXERCISE ONE**

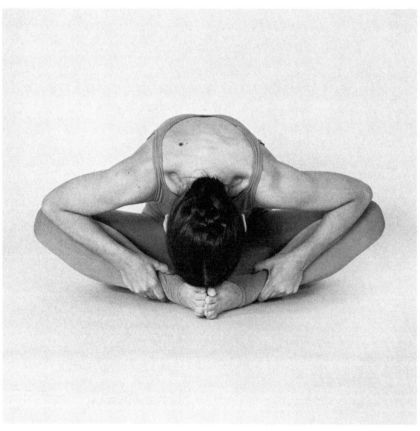

nant). If you can't get your knees down on the floor—one of the most important factors in the exercise—practice by putting the soles of your feet together and pushing your knees down with your hands (Fig. 10–15). If you do this about ten minutes a day, your knees will be on the floor in a couple of months.

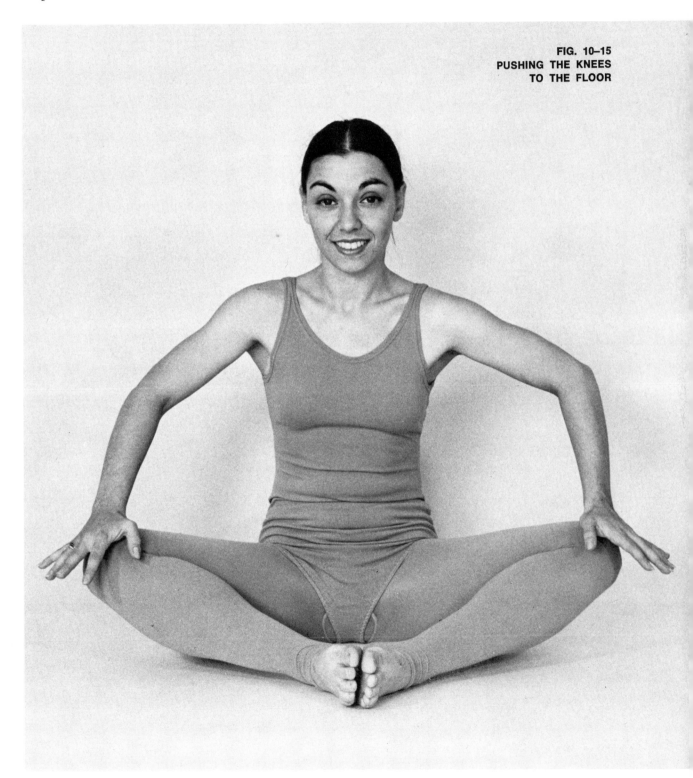

**FIG. 10–15
PUSHING THE KNEES
TO THE FLOOR**

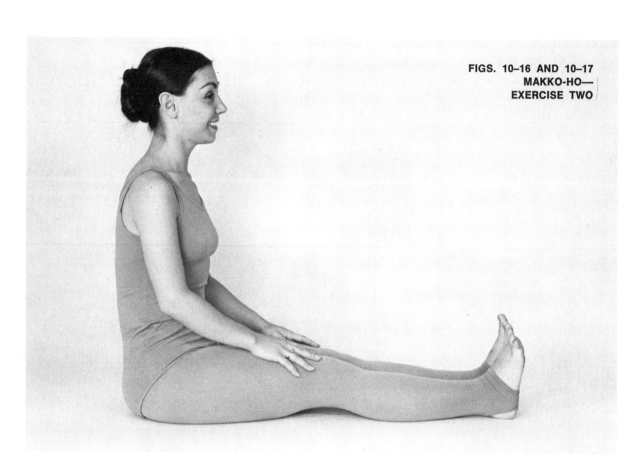

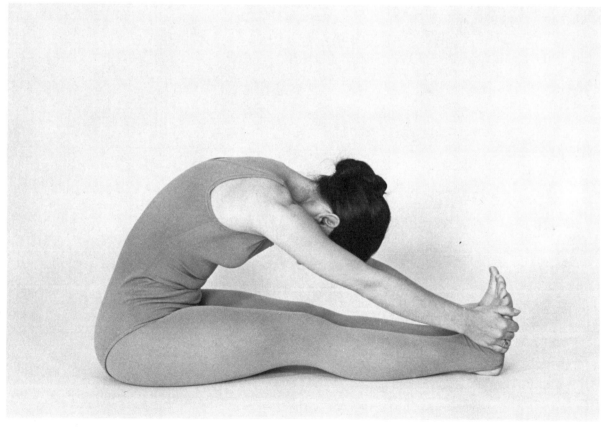

126

EXERCISE TWO

Sit up with a straight back and stretch both your legs in front of you. Keep your feet flexed at a 60-degree angle. Now bend your body forward and grab the soles of your feet without bending your knees (Figs. 10–16 and 10–17). Do this ten or twenty times. If you can't get close enough to your feet to grab them, go as far forward as possible without bending your knees. This exercise stretches the muscles in the Achilles tendon, the ankle, and on the back side of the legs. Again, not for pregnant women.

EXERCISE THREE

Open your legs to a 180-degree angle and extending your arms forward, bend your body so your head touches the floor. Do this ten or twenty times. This will improve flexibility in the sockets of the leg joints and in the muscles. This increased flexibility can lead to a happier sex life and can regulate menstrual problems and frigidity. Unlike the first two Makko-Ho exercises, this one is good to do if you are pregnant; it will improve your chances for an easy delivery (Fig. 10–18).

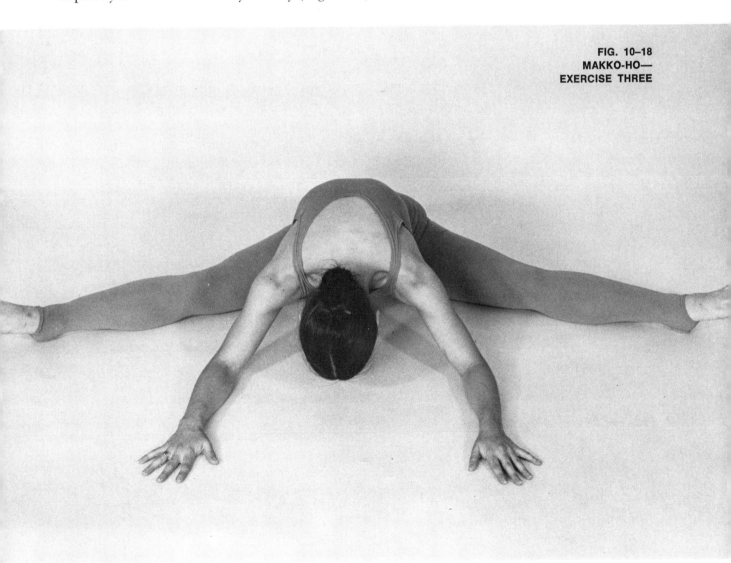

**FIG. 10–18
MAKKO-HO—
EXERCISE THREE**

EXERCISE FOUR

Sit on your heels with a straight back (Fig. 10–19). Relax. This is the traditional Japanese sitting posture for women and is also used in Zen meditation. Leaving your feet where they are, lie down backward, keeping your hips on the floor and your knees as close together as possible. Avoid arching your back or allowing your knees to spread. Stay there for a couple of minutes, breathing deeply and steadily (Fig. 10–20). If your buttocks are not on the floor in the sitting position you may place a cushion beneath them, and if it is difficult to bend all the way back, place a low piece of furniture behind you and lean on that. This exercise stretches the back and can correct a forward bend in the lumbar vertebrae.

FIGS. 10–19 AND 10–20 MAKKO-HO— EXERCISE FOUR

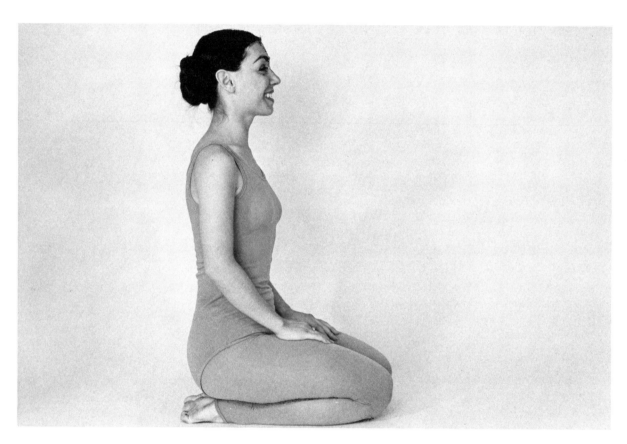

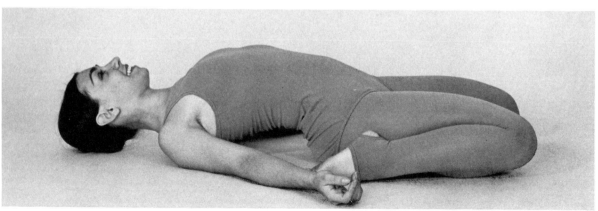

Swinging and Rocking

Here are two final exercises you can do yourself which greatly benefit the spine.

SWINGING EXERCISES

Stand up with your legs open in a comfortable position. Spreading your arms wide, rotate your body to the right and the left. Don't force yourself; relax and swing comfortably. Don't twist your feet. Do this for two or three minutes. Continue rotating your torso, but now, for a more extreme stretch, swing your leg up in the opposite direction of your torso. When the torso rotates to the left, your leg swings up to the right (Fig. 10–21). Let your arms go. Swing both legs. You may hear your lumbar vertebrae cracking. Both these exercises are good for the lower back and relax back muscles.

FIG. 10–21
SWINGING EXERCISE

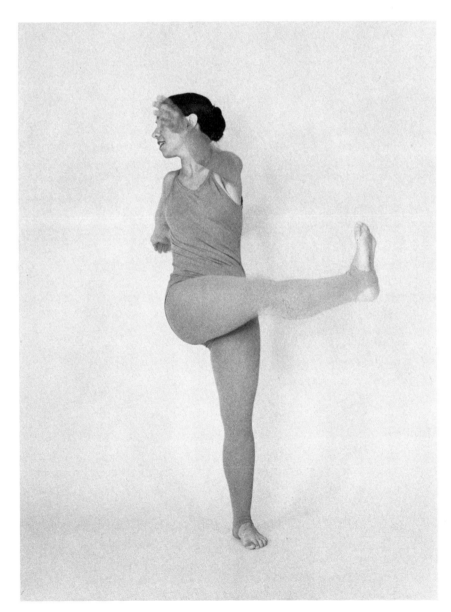

ROCKING EXERCISE

Sit up straight with your legs crossed and grab each foot with the corresponding hand. Tuck your chin and rock backward, then up and forward again. For best results your body should be relaxed. This exercise, done for five minutes two or three times a day, makes your spine more flexible because your own weight rocking massages it (Fig. 10–22).

**FIG. 10–22
ROCKING EXERCISE**

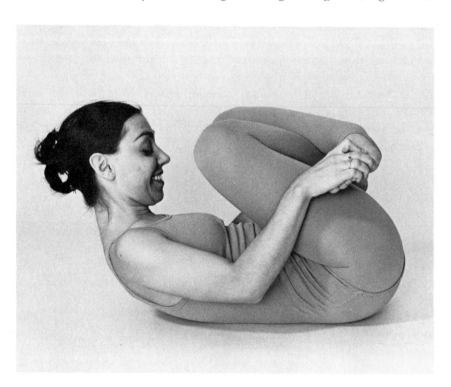

11. General Shiatsu and How to Treat Common Ailments with Shiatsu

Congratulations! You have now learned the fundamental techniques of Shiatsu—a skill which will make you a great benefactor to your friends and family members. As you give Shiatsu treatments to those closest to you, you will become more sensitive to their bodies and feelings than ever before. Giving Shiatsu to strangers will inevitably make you friends—you will be opening your communication on a level which goes beyond and deeper than anything you could say in words. Of course, you are still not an expert, but the more you practice Shiatsu the faster you will be able to locate tsubos, the more penetrating your fingers will become, and the better you will understand the human body and the pain and pleasure you can give it with your fingers.

Giving Shiatsu to the Entire Body

In order to cultivate the health of your patient's body you must give him general Shiatsu—or Shiatsu that stimulates all the meridian lines. Even if he or she is suffering from a single, specific ailment, you should give general Shiatsu, because no health problem exists in isolation but indicates a stagnation or slowdown in energy throughout the body. By now you have studied the processes for giving Shiatsu to the back, Hara, neck, limbs, and head. I will now give you a routine for general Shiatsu and tell the order in which you can apply the techniques you have already learned.

1. Back Shiatsu. Ask the patient to lie on his stomach and relax. Warm up his back before you start pressing specific tsubos. Using your fingers, thumbs, and palms practice Kenbiki, or pushing and pulling the muscles. Find out where he has stiffness, temperature, and pain. Apply the special techniques described in chapter 3 when they are appropriate. Then press the tsubos on the Bladder Meridian, from Bladder #11 to #26. Repeat three times. Then press Bladder #41 to #52. Repeat three times.

2. While the patient is on his stomach, give Shiatsu to the hips and the backs of the legs.

131

3. Give Shiatsu to the feet.
4. Ask the patient to lie on his back. Give Ampuku.
5. Give Shiatsu to the front of the legs.
6. Give Shiatsu to the chest and arms.
7. Give Shiatsu to the neck, head, and face.
8. Have the patient sit up. Give Shiatsu to the back of the neck, head, and shoulders.

The entire routine should take from thirty minutes to one hour. If your patient has a particular problem, concentrate on the tsubos used to treat it after giving general Shiatsu. As you become more experienced and learn to know your patient's body, you will develop and apply the techniques that are most helpful to that individual.

How to Treat Common Ailments

On the following pages I have selected a number of diseases, ailments, and chronic health problems, listed them in alphabetical order and described how to relieve them with Shiatsu. Shiatsu may not cure these problems permanently, but it can alleviate their symptoms if applied regularly and properly. Of course I have not been able to include every ailment known to man, nor have I repeated every treatment described in the preceding chapters. I have limited the tsubos used to treat ailments to those described in chapter 2. If you are unsure about the location of a tsubo or how to press it, you should consult chapter 2 and my chart. In some cases I have recommended pressing a particular tsubo that is not directly related to a particular ailment. These are tsubos which indirectly affect the problem; which increase the body's total output of energy needed to fight the disease; or which work in conjunction with the other tsubos I have asked you to press.

In many cases I have also recommended dietary remedies or described a disease and its cause according to the principles of Oriental medicine.

ARTHRITIS

We are not yet sure what causes arthritis, the common disease whose worst symptom is a painful and restricting inflammation of the joints. It may be an excess of toxins in the body or too much humidity in the atmosphere. To help ease arthritic pain, push and pull the muscles in the area where the pain is most intense and give general Shiatsu to that area. Then press the following tsubos: Bladder #20 and #25 and Conception Vessel #6.

ASTHMA

No one knows exactly what causes asthma, either. People with allergies tend to develop it, and air pollution, weather, and diets that include too much animal protein, sugar, and overly spiced foods may be contributing factors. You can relieve asthma symptoms with the following treatments:
1. Give neck Shiatsu. Give Shiatsu to both sides of the neck because

asthmatic coughing makes the muscles in these areas tight and stiff. Asthma or any lung problem will also create pain in the back and shoulders, so give Shiatsu to these parts of the body. (See chapter 4.)

2. Press in below the rib cage as patient breathes out. (See pp. 106–107.)

3. Press the following tsubos: Bladder #12 and #13, Lung #1, and Gall Bladder #21.

4. Massage treatment: Take a dry towel and rub the extremities of the body, working your way toward the heart. Continue until the body feels hot. The dry-towel massage promotes good circulation and skin respiration, and strengthens the skin; it improves the health of the whole body. Do it out of doors in the fresh air if possible, even in winter.

BALDING

To retard or prevent balding by stimulating hair follicles, massage the scalp with your fingers, give neck Shiatsu, pressing Governing Vessel #14 and Gall Bladder #20 to give good circulation and soften the skin of the scalp. Then give general Shiatsu to the head and face, pressing and massaging the Governing Vessel, Bladder, and Gall Bladder meridians. You can apply this treatment to your own head, four or five times a day.

BED-WETTING

I was a bed-wetter until the age of ten. My father shamed me by scolding me in front of my sisters. It seemed the more I tried to stop, the more nervous I became and the more I wet the bed. My mother, a wise woman, gave me general Shiatsu and Ampuku and my bed-wetting problem stopped at once. Nervous children are prone to bed-wetting, and when they are scolded for it, the problem becomes worse. It has been found that children who are chronic bed-wetters often have some bone structure distortion and abnormal stiffness in the back and sides of the body. Here are some exercises and Shiatsu techniques to stop bed-wetting:

1. Place the child on his back. Stretch and open both his legs. Pinch each of his toes with your thumb and index finger and then pull them gently. Massage each toe for two or three minutes. Pinch his big toe with your thumb and index finger; still holding the toe, raise his leg until the toe is two inches away from the child's head. Shake the leg by the toe. Repeat this with each toe.

2. In Japan we tickle bed-wetters, but only with a playful attitude and if the child enjoys it. Lock the child's head between your knees and tickle him on both sides of the torso. As he laughs he will tend to twist his body to the opposite side of the one you are tickling, which helps correct curvatures or malformations of the body's structure. Tickle for two to five minutes.

3. Give Shiatsu to Ten Shi, along the sacrum, pressing the four grooves on each side, on the side of the neck and especially on Bladder #10. Press the first line of tsubos on the Bladder Meridian along the spine.

4. Give Ampuku.

BLEMISHES

See chapter 9.

COLITIS

If you do not know why you have colitis, or spastic colon, be sure to be checked by a physician; colitis is caused by a very critical problem with the internal organs. To relieve symptoms with Shiatsu, press Bladder Meridian tsubos #18, #19, #21, #25, and #27; give neck Shiatsu, chest Shiatsu, and Ampuku, pinching the muscles around the navel gently.

COMMON COLD

There is a Japanese proverb which says "the cold leads to all diseases." This means that a cold, if left untreated, can cause more serious problems. To prevent colds, try to maintain a diet that is low on sweets, especially chocolate, take vitamin C, get sun, and give yourself the dry-towel massage, described above under "Asthma."

The best treatment for a cold is to rest the body and mind, keep warm, and take natural vitamin C. Easily digestible protein promotes energy in the body which fights the cold. To treat colds, give general Shiatsu first. Then press Bladder #10, #12, and #13, Gall Bladder #20, and Large Intestine #4 and #11 to ease aches, pains, and other symptoms and increase bodily energy. See chapter 9 for techniques to relieve nasal stagnation; also see "Headaches" and "Sinus Congestion" in this listing.

CONSTIPATION

Constipation is a chronic American ailment, especially among young women. It is a more dangerous problem than you might think, more harmful than diarrhea, because it causes toxins to spread through the body and affect other organs. Some of the side effects of constipation are headache, dizziness, insomnia, skin blemishes, cancer, poor circulation, colitis, lower-back ache, shoulder pain, fatigue, and early deterioration, to name a few. Some causes of constipation are nervous tension, mental stress, disorder of autonomic nervous system, postponing bowel movements, problems in the digestive tract, sexual organ malfunctions, pregnancy, lack of exercise, stomach cancer, lack of vegetables (especially fibrous vegetables) in the diet, and overeating.

To cure constipation, change your diet first. You should eat raw vegetables, including fibrous ones such as cabbage and apples, brown rice, and soybeans. You must flood your body with liquids to enable it to wash wastes away. Water mixed with sea kelp before breakfast is a helpful remedy. Sometimes a complete fast detoxifies your intestines and gives them a rest. Make it part of your daily routine to visit the toilet each morning, or whenever you feel like it; don't postpone. Exercise is also important. Move, but relax. Never, under any circumstances, should you take drugstore laxatives. They weaken your body and make constipation worse.

Give general Shiatsu. Give Kenbiki along the Bladder Meridian, especially in places where stiffness is felt. Just above the hipbones on each side of the body, about one inch above Ten Shi, there is a tsubo (not listed in chapter 2) which we call the "constipation point." Press hard and inward on both of these points for 5–7 seconds, four or five times. Give soft Ampuku to the upper Hara, and a little stronger Ampuku to the lower Hara. The descending colon, in the left side of the Hara, must be treated gently. If you are a constipation victim you should give yourself Ampuku with your legs bent for 10–15 minutes every morning in bed before you get up.

Press the following tsubos: Conception Vessel #6, Bladder #23, #25, #32, Stomach #36, Large Intestine #4 (if you are constipated this point will be painful), and Ohashi's point in the neck.

The Makko-Ho exercises in chapter 10 are also helpful. Really stretch your legs when you are doing them—especially the left leg.

DIABETES

The best way to relieve the symptoms of diabetes is to follow the diet your doctor recommends. Shiatsu cannot cure diabetes, but general Shiatsu on the whole body, pressing the Associated Points on the Bladder Meridian (Bladder #20, #19, #18, and #23), and Ampuku therapy can stimulate the function of the pancreas, liver, and their associated organs.

DIARRHEA

Diarrhea is one of the ways the body rids itself of poisonous or spoiled foods: (Vomiting is another way the body ejects dangerous intruders.) It can also be caused by overeating, nervous tension, anxiety, obsession, colds, flu (Lung Meridian malfunctions also cause Large Intestine problems), general weaknesses of the system, and a weak or cold Hara. A cold that causes pain in the back or legs will certainly be accompanied by diarrhea. Some kinds of diarrhea, like dysentery, are caused by infectious parasites in the intestines and should be treated by a professional.

Diarrhea is most dangerous in babies because it rapidly drains their small bodies of fluids. As a small child I nearly died of diarrhea. At that time, right after the war, Japan had no hospitals or medicine; my father fortunately took me to a folk medicine doctor who treated my back and stomach with Moxa. I owe my life to him.

When you get diarrhea you can fast for a couple of days to detoxify your digestive system. Be sure to replace lost liquids with teas; herb teas, especially sage tea, are good for toning the stomach and stopping diarrhea. Diarrhea may be the result of a chill in the Hara; warm it by wrapping four or five recently hard-boiled eggs in a towel (the eggs hold heat for a long time) and place them on your Hara, rubbing it. Give Kenbiki to the Bladder Meridian in the back and then press the following tsubos: Ten Shi, Stomach #34 and #36, Kidney #1, and Conception Vessel #6 and #12. Give very gentle Shiatsu to the lower Hara, and slightly stronger Shiatsu to the upper Hara. Don't forget general Ampuku. Press the grooves on both sides of the sacrum.

DIZZINESS

Keep the dizzy patient quiet. Give him neck Shiatsu and press Large Intestine #4, Liver #3, Kidney #1, and In Do.

EPILEPSY

Those who have a tendency for epilepsy can encourage it by eating acid foods like animal protein products (meat, milk, cheese, etc.). According to Oriental theory of diet, these foods are Yang and should be balanced by Yin foods (grains, vegetable protein, and green vegetables).

Food poisoning, fried foods, and lack of calcium can also bring on seizures in the potential epileptic.

If you are near someone who has an epileptic seizure, remain calm and do not act upset or shocked. Lower his body temperature by removing his clothing and keep him cool. Quickly stuff a wadded handkerchief in his mouth, under his tongue, to prevent him from biting it. Make sure there is plenty of ventilation—preferably cool, dry air. Place a wet towel on his head.

Press the Bladder Meridian along the spine and Governing Vessel #14, #25, and #26; Bladder #60 (pinch Bladder #60 and the other side of the foot together); Conception Vessel #12; and Kidney #1. Press hard on the Achilles tendon; pinch the big toe with your thumb and index finger, and press hard on his palms.

EYE PROBLEMS

When you were a child your mother probably told you not to rub your eyes with your hands. Actually, it is good to rub and stimulate the eyes, carefully, of course, and with clean hands. (See eye massages in chapter 9.) If your eyes feel hot, place a chilled towel on them. After a few minutes remove it and rub your eyes gently with the towel. If you are reading a great deal and your eyes become tired, try looking far off into the distance with relaxed eyes. Do not strain to see anything, just gaze into the distance once every hour. An eye exercise to relax and strengthen the eyes goes like this: center your eyes in the middle, then look up and down slowly and return your eyes to center. Stretch your eyes as far as they will go without strain. Do the same looking left and right, diagonally, and rolling your eyes clockwise and counterclockwise. Rotate your neck slowly. Then press Sei Mei, or Bladder #1, rolling your index finger toward the nose. The eyes should be closed. You can also press gently along the bone that encircles the eyes.

For tired eyes, near-sightedness, and far-sightedness, press the following points: Tai Yo, Bladder #20, the center of each eyebrow, and Large Intestine #4.

People with eye problems and chronically tired eyes always complain of pain in the neck, back, and shoulders. These pains can be alleviated by pressing Gall Bladder #21, Bladder #20, Governing Vessel #14, and Ohashi's point between the third and fourth cervical vertebrae in the neck. Remember, according to the philosophy of Oriental medicine, the eyes are the mirror of the liver and the liver requires vitamin A to function well. Avoid excessive amounts of oil, fats, and don't overeat.

FAINTING AND LOSS OF CONSCIOUSNESS

Fainting can be serious if loss of consciousness continues for an extended period of time. If breathing stops, the patient can die. If fainting is due to hysteria or shock, the patient usually recovers if left alone. A slap or water splashed in his face can help too. If loss of consciousness is due to drowning or heart attack, press Conception Vessel #1 (not on the chart in chapter 2 but located in the perineum, between the anus and the genitals) with an instrument like a dull hairpin (do not puncture the skin). (See "Heart Attack" for further information.)

FATIGUE

For fatigue, give general Shiatsu and then Ampuku, especially on the Tan Den point to stimulate revitalizing life-sexual energy. Give neck Shiatsu and press Governing Vessel #14, Gall Bladder #20 and #21. If fatigue is chronic, the liver and pancreas may be malfunctioning as well as other organs, and you should see a physician.

FRIGIDITY

If a woman is frigid or has no desire for sex her lover should help by giving her general Shiatsu with gentle love and affection every day, especially before going to bed. He also should press Bladder Meridian tsubos #23, #26, and #27, Stomach #9, and give Shiatsu to the front of the neck and thyroid area. Ampuku is also important to increase sexual energy. (See "Sexual Stamina" below, for increasing sexual energy in both men and women.)

HEADACHES (see also "Migraine Headaches")

When I was working as a Shiatsu therapist at the Watergate Health Club in Washington, D.C., I treated some very painful headaches among politicians, ambassadors, and government officials. As the Watergate case became more notorious the headaches increased.

Headache is such a common ailment that everyone suffers from it at least once in his life. But we still find it hard to say exactly what causes each headache to occur, since there are at least 140 reasons why we suffer head pain. Usually headache is connected with some sort of muscle tension; contraction of tense muscles causes spasms in the blood vessels that run through them; circulation is obstructed and the symptom is discomfort in the brain area. Muscle tension is caused by a hectic, busy life; by noise, anxiety, and stress. If you keep the same position for a long time, when you drive a car or type, for example, your neck muscles become tight with tension. Other causes of headache are insomnia, uremic poisoning, tuberculosis, allergy, nasal congestion, toothache, and whiplash.

There are many ways to cure chronic headache. First, relax and change your approach to life. Things will happen as they may whether you worry about them or not. Exercise. Correct your posture if you have a lazy or bent spine. Make sure your diet includes sufficient vitamins A and C. Avoid sugar, beef, and refined flours and grains. Do *not* take aspirin. Pain is nature's signal that something is wrong. Try to get to the source of the problem. Aspirin destroys vitamin C and irritates the stomach lining.

To treat a headache, put your left hand on the patient's forehead. Give neck Shiatsu with your right hand, pressing the forehead for five minutes. Give head, shoulder, and upper-back Shiatsu, and massage the part of the head where there is pain. Give Shiatsu to the temples and Tai Yo point. You can treat yourself this way as well as your patient. If you know the underlying cause for the headache, treat that first and then the headache symptoms. Pressing the following tsubos will relieve headache pain: Governing Vessel #11 and #15, Stomach #36, Gall Bladder #20 and #21, Bladder #10, #13, and #60, Large Intestine #4 and #11, Liver #3, and In Do.

HEART ATTACK

If someone has a heart attack, practice *Katsu*—that is, put one bent knee on the patient's heart point area, Bladder #15, and thrust with the knee while pulling up the patient's right shoulder and pulling down his left shoulder. Pull the little finger. Then stretch your arms and press the heart repeatedly, using your weight, keeping the patient on his back. Press Kidney #1, Lung #9, Heart #7, and Governing Vessel #26. Pinch and press hard on the big toe.

HEMORRHOIDS

Strong liquor, seasoned food, constipation, and overeating cause liver malfunctions. A malfunctioning liver increases blood pressure in the veins, which in turn causes them to swell painfully in the anus. You can massage the anus yourself in the bath, or by cleaning your fingers and moistening them with good quality vegetable oil. Gently press the swollen and distended parts of the anus back into place. Press hard on the following points: Bladder #18, #23, #25, #26, Governing Vessel #9 (on the spine between the seventh and eighth thoracic vertebrae) and #20. If constipation is the cause of your hemorrhoids treat that problem as well. (See "Constipation" in this listing.)

HICCUPS

We don't know exactly what causes hiccups but they are common, and an extended attack can cause much suffering. To stop hiccups, first press Conception Vessel #22 (not on the chart; located in the soft depression between the two collarbones), then Stomach #9, Bladder #15 and #17. Press closed eyes very gently with your fingers and drink a glass of water just before the next hiccup.

HIGH BLOOD PRESSURE (HYPERTENSION)

High blood pressure is caused by overeating, too much salt, animal protein, drinking, and smoking. Kidney problems, thyroid problems, hormone malfunction, arteriosclerosis, nervous tension, and overwork are all related to high blood pressure. Heredity, too, may be a factor for some people who have this problem. High blood pressure can cause brain damage, headache, dizziness, insomnia, shoulder pain, heart problems and palpitations, constipation, kidney trouble, and ringing in the ears.

To treat high blood pressure with Shiatsu, press Large Intestine #11, Stomach #9 and #36, Kidney #1, Bladder #15 and #22, and Gall Bladder #21. Stomach #9 is especially excellent for this problem. Pull the middle and little fingers. Give general Shiatsu softly for twenty or thirty minutes. Ampuku is essential when high blood pressure is accompanied by constipation. Give neck Shiatsu. If the patient's blood pressure is over 200, don't give Shiatsu at all.

IMPOTENCE

For impotence in men, press Conception Vessel #1 (see "Sexual Stamina," below, for its location) and #4 (Kan Gen), Spleen #6,

Stomach #36, and Bladder #23. General Shiatsu and Ampuku should be given by a loving partner.

INSOMNIA

Human beings need a certain amount of sleep every night. Deprivation can lead to mental disorders and even death. Sleep comes naturally unless we are somehow resisting it (through tension, emotional stress, etc.). The insomniac finds himself caught in a vicious circle. He worries because he can't sleep, which leads to further tension, which increases his insomnia; the more he believes he is a hopeless insomniac the more he worries about it, and so on. In some cases of insomnia the patient does need medical or psychological help. In general, though, the insomniac should not force himself into an unnatural sleep cycle, but involve himself in other activities until sleep overtakes him.

To prevent insomnia, guard against body pain or itching, mental or emotional stress, fever, too much coffee or tea. Do not eat or drink too much before retiring; if your internal organs are still working to digest your dinner, a deep, relaxed sleep is impossible.

Here is a Shiatsu treatment for insomnia: Give general Shiatsu first. Press Tai Yo. Give neck Shiatsu, pressing the Ohashi point. Give Shiatsu along the Bladder Meridian, especially to Bladder #25. Press Kidney #1 and give foot Shiatsu. Give Ampuku. Press Spleen #6 and Governing Vessel #20. Sex can help insomnia because it relaxes the muscles of the body. Do *not* take sleeping pills—they only make insomnia worse. Exercise every day. Take a walk. Change your diet to include alkaline foods. Take vitamin B complex, sunbathe and swim in the ocean if you can. Saltwater and sun are a relaxing combination.

LABOR

To ease pain before delivery, give Shiatsu to Bladder #32, Spleen #6, and the tsubos on the sacrum; massage the end of the sacrum, or tailbone. Give gentle Ampuku during pregnancy.

LACTATION

Mother's milk is the best food for your baby. If you don't have enough milk, the following Shiatsu procedures should improve lactation. Press Gall Bladder #21; trace the rib cage as described in chapter 8. Then warm your hands and place your palms on the breasts, rotating in clockwise direction gently.

LOWER-BACK ACHE

The lower back supports the Hara and sustains the weight of our bodies —a difficult and demanding job. Animals do not get lower-back ache because they do not walk upright, and their weight does not fall onto only one part of the back. Statistics show that over six million Americans suffer from this ailment, which troubles comparatively few Japanese. Why? Americans tend to overeat and eat the wrong foods. Their excess fat adds a heavy load to the lumbar of the lower back. Almost everyone in this country has a car and seldom walks. This causes weak legs which cannot support the back properly. Lack of exercise, in general, makes the back weak too. Americans sleep on soft beds which cause the body to shrink and sag with the bed, contracting muscles and stagnating the blood—the result is lower-back ache. I've noticed that the person who eats refined, mushy foods, sweet desserts, fancy sauces, and drinks a lot seems to be the same kind of person who sleeps on a soft, mushy, refined bed and suffers from lower-back ache. Japanese, on the other hand, prefer to sleep on a slim cotton mattress called *futon* which they spread on a hard rice mat, or tatami.

There are also mechanical reasons for lower-back ache, including overwork, muscle fatigue, a sudden twist, cold weather, or broken bones. Pains from malfunctioning internal organs also show up in the lower back, shoulders, and neck.

Prevention is the best cure for lower-back ache. But if you get a lower-back ache, stay quiet and rest; do not move your body. Lie on your side and bend your body so it is shaped like a shrimp; this is the most comfortable sleeping position for lower-back ache. Keep your back warm. Hot pads, bottles, and towels promote blood circulation and make Shiatsu treatment more effective.

To treat backache with Shiatsu, first find the location of the pain. Is it in the upper or lower back, right or left side? Is it superficial or deep? After you have diagnosed, give a rubdown and Kenbiki, not Shiatsu, on the *opposite* side from the side where there is pain. Work from the shoulder to the hip and the thigh to the calf, then repeat the treatment from the shoulder on the painful side to the calf. Then begin pressing the tsubos where the patient feels pain. I have found that lower-back ache is often centered between the fourth and fifth lumbar vertebrae, especially on the left side, in Bladder #25. Give Shiatsu to this tsubo if you find pain there. Other points to press for lower-back ache are Bladder #26, #27, #28, #29, #30, #36, #52, and Ten Shi. If you want to treat your own backache, sit with crossed legs in the lotus position and press these points on your own spine with your thumbs.

Shiatsu treatment is most effective the moment lower-back ache pain begins. If the pain has its origin in the internal organs, it will be more difficult to cure. If lower-back ache is accompanied by diarrhea and menstrual cramps, give Ampuku therapy. Lower-back ache can also give severe pain in the Ohashi point on the neck.

Do not give Shiatsu for lower-back ache when there are broken bones, TB of the spine, a slipped disk, or bone diseases, especially when the person is taking cortisone or its derivatives.

Many doctors recommend surgery for chronic lower-back ache. In my opinion, surgery on the lower back is such a complicated and dangerous procedure that no one should subject himself to it. There are delicate nerves in the spinal cord; if they are upset or damaged, the ability to walk or stand can be endangered and the lower part of the body could become paralyzed. You have to prevent your lower-back problems.

MENOPAUSE

Symptoms of menopause appear throughout the body. Many women experience headaches, insomnia, constipation, loss or gain of weight. They feel that their entire body function is changing and this can lead to emotional stress and upset. Give the patient general Shiatsu for twenty or thirty minutes, neck Shiatsu, and sacrum Shiatsu. Press Spleen #6 and #10, Bladder #23 and #47 to increase energy in the circulatory system.

MENSTRUAL PAIN

It is hard to understand why some women suffer unbearable menstrual pain while others have none at all. Pressing the following points can relieve these monthly agonies: Spleen #6 and #10, Bladder #23 and #32. Stimulating these tsubos helps to eliminate stagnation of blood circulation which causes the pain. Ampuku should be given too.

MIGRAINE HEADACHES

Migraines occur regularly and are an especially fearful form of headache, totally disabling the patient. If you suffer from migraine on one side of the head, you will also have pain and stiffness in the neck and shoulder on that side. Sometimes that side of the back is affected too. Give Shiatsu to the neck, shoulder, and back on the painful side; this also relieves head pain.

To relieve migraine you must first discover which meridian malfunction is causing it. If migraine pain is in the front of the head, it may be due to a malfunction of the Stomach and Lung meridians. Treat it by giving Shiatsu along those meridians, and pressing Tai Yo, Bladder #21, and Stomach #36. Migraines on the side of the head are probably due to a malfunction of the Gall Bladder Meridian. I have found that there is usually more pain on the left side. Give Shiatsu along the Gall Bladder Meridian. Since Gall Bladder #1, next to the eyes, is usually too painful to touch, begin working on Gall Bladder points on the back of the neck and work your way forward to Gall Bladder #1. Concentrate on Gall Bladder #20, #21, and Bladder #19. Migraines in the back of the head indicate a malfunction of the Bladder Meridian. Give Shiatsu mainly along the Bladder Meridian line, especially Bladder #10, #23, and #60. Press Ohashi's point (very important) and Governing Vessel #14.

NEURALGIA

Neuralgia pain, originating in an inflamed nerve, can occur anywhere in the body. People with an acid or Yang diet (lots of animal products) have a greater tendency to get neuralgia. Cold and mental strain also affect those with a tendency for this problem. To treat neuralgia, give Shiatsu to the whole body; this circulates the blood through the nerves and provides nerves and muscles with oxygen and ventilation. Then concentrate on the area where there is pain. Give neck Shiatsu.

NOSEBLEED

Try the following treatment for nosebleed. Press Large Intestine #20, Bladder #10, and Governing Vessel #14. Press both sides of each toe strongly and give neck Shiatsu.

RINGING IN THE EARS

Ringing in the ears may be due to a kidney problem if the cause is not mechanical. Press Gall Bladder #2 and #17, Bladder #23 and #52, Triple Heater #17 and #21. Give general Shiatsu to the area around the ears.

SCIATICA

For sciatica, or pain radiating down the legs, give Shiatsu to the side with pain. Press Bladder #23, #36, #52, and the following points in the legs: Bladder #40, Bladder #37, Bladder #60, Gall Bladder #31, and Stomach #36. Also press Gall Bladder #30 and Ten Shi. The first and second exercises for two described in chapter 10 will also relieve sciatic pain.

SEXUAL STAMINA

A happy sex life depends on good health throughout the body. If a couple practices Shiatsu, each member will give the other a way to gain good health and love in the form of personal touching. I have found that people who have a poor sex life have a tight back and Hara. The hips, back, and Hara must be soft and flexible for a good sex life. Pressing the Bladder Meridian along the spine is one of the best ways to promote general health and a happy sex life along with it. Bladder points #18, #19, #20, #23, #24, #26, and #52 and Spleen #6 are especially important. Pushing and pulling the muscles on the back with your fingers (Kenbiki) is also useful. Pressing the tsubos on both sides of the sacrum (Bladder #31, #32, #33, and #34) directly stimulates the sex organs. Press hard and inward. Finally, be sure to practice Ampuku on yourself and your sexual partner regularly.

Women with weak thighs (on the insides) are often weak sexually. Ask the patient to lie on her back and place your open palms on the insides of her thighs and press down gently, gradually applying your body weight, for 7–10 seconds. If she feels pain and has little strength on the insides of her thighs her sexual energy may be low. To strengthen her thigh and groin region and improve its flexibility, have her lie on her back and continue the preceding exercise regularly. For variation you can place one of her legs, bent at the knee, on top of the other and press the insides of her thighs outward.

Conception Vessel #1, not shown on the chart in chapter 2, is located in the perineum, between the genitals and the anus. Give Shiatsu on this point for 5–7 minutes to stimulate the sex function directly. Tan Den Ampuku (Conception Vessel #4) is also necessary.

SINUS CONGESTION

For stagnation and congestion in the nose, press the following points: Governing Vessel #14, Large Intestine #4 and #20, Stomach #6, and Bladder #20. Nose stagnation is a symptom of Lung and Large Intestine meridian malfunction (like constipation) and can be caused by overeating, especially before going to bed.

SORE THROAT

To relieve sore throat symptoms, press Lung #11, Large Intestine #4, and Stomach #9.

STIFF NECK

Stiff necks are sometimes caused by high blood pressure and lower-back ache, toothache, and nervous tension. Treat the underlying cause if you can. Give neck Shiatsu, back Shiatsu, and Kenbiki on the back, chest, and arms. Heat is helpful. Rotate the neck.

STOMACH CRAMPS

To relieve cramps, give neck Shiatsu, especially in the Ohashi point, and press Bladder #21, #22, and #50 (one and a half inches to the side of Bladder #21), and Stomach #34. Give Ampuku in the upper Hara, around the navel, and under the rib cage. Place your palm on the navel and rotate slowly. Give Kenbiki to the back.

STOMACH SPASM

Give strong Shiatsu to Bladder #17 and #18, Stomach #34, Liver #3; also give gentle Ampuku.

SWALLOWING DIFFICULTY

If you are having trouble swallowing due to obstruction in the throat or deterioration from old age, take chest Shiatsu as described in chapter 8. Press Conception Vessel #17 and Governing Vessel #13.

TOOTHACHE

Shiatsu relieves the pain of toothache only temporarily. You should see a dentist as soon as possible. Press the points where you have pain and Tai Yo, Large Intestine #4 (used in Acupuncture to anesthetize the gums), Large Intestine #10, and Stomach #3. Massage the gums regularly to improve circulation and strengthen the roots. This kind of Shiatsu is especially good for preventing pyorrhea. Neck Shiatsu is helpful.

VOMITING

There are many reasons why we are induced to vomit:

1. Motion sickness, often encouraged by overeating and drinking in combination with a nervous stomach, or an imbalance in the ear mechanisms.

2. Poisoned food. When you ingest poison your body tries to reject it. This is a healthy sign; your body is protecting you and you should be happy to vomit. If you cannot, try the following remedy: Take three teaspoons of salt in a cup of warm water, or rice vinegar instead of salt if it is available. Then place your index finger or toothbrush inside down the back of your throat and massage.

3. Pregnancy. During pregnancy there may be a good deal of nausea and desire to vomit, because there is a new addition to the Hara area to which the body is not accustomed. A good remedy for this problem is eating *umeboshi*, a sour plum, which you can buy in a Japanese grocery store. It will improve the appetite and has a delightful flavor.

4. Appendicitis and kidney stone. If you have one of these problems, you will, of course, need surgery.

5. During illness accompanied by fever and chills. Again this is your

body's attempt to rid itself of toxins and mucus. You should not eat solid foods; drink fruit juice instead.

To treat extreme or undue vomiting give Kenbiki on the back along the Bladder Meridian, Ampuku therapy, and neck Shiatsu.